Child Development Mediated by Trauma

T0383617

Drawing on clinical data obtained through the study of children adopted from overseas orphanages, the author of this cutting-edge text applies the Developmental Trauma Disorder (DTD) conceptual framework to the analysis of psychological, educational, and mental health impact of the early childhood trauma on development of internationally adopted children.

A massive scale of international adoption of children, victims of profound neglect and deprivation, combined with the fundamental change in a child's social situation of development after adoption, offers a valuable opportunity to explore the concept of Developmental Trauma Disorder: developmental delays, emotional vulnerability, "mixed maturity," cumulative cognitive deficit, and post-orphanage behavior patterns, being presented by many adoptees long after the adoption. By focusing on the neurological and psychological nature of childhood trauma, Dr. Gindis offers a unique approach to understanding the ongoing impacts of DTD and the ways in which any subsequent neuropsychological, educational, and mental health issues might be assessed.

This book will be of great interest to researchers in the fields of psychology, mental health, education, and child development; as well as clinicians involved in trauma treatment and international adoption.

Boris Gindis is licensed psychologist, USA.

Explorations in Developmental Psychology

Developmental Neuropsychology
Janna Glozman

Indigenous Adolescent Development
Psychological, Social and Historical Contexts
Les B. Whitbeck, Kelley J. Sittner Hartshorn and Melissa L. Walls

Learning from Picturebooks
Research from Cognitive Psychology, Early Literacy, and
Child Developmental Studies
Edited by Bettina Kummerling-Meibauer, Jörg Meibauer,
Kerstin Nachtigäller and Katharina Rohlfing

Development from Adolescence to Early Adulthood
A Dynamic Systemic Approach to Transitions and Transformations
Marion Kloep, Leo B. Hendry, Rachel Taylor and Ian Stuart-Hamilton

Teachers, Learners, Modes of Practice
Theory and Methodology for Identifying Knowledge Development
David Kirk Dirlam

Children's Books, Brain Development, and Language Acquisition
Ralf Thiede

Child Development Mediated by Trauma
The Dark Side of International Adoption
Boris Gindis

Child Development Mediated by Trauma

The Dark Side of International Adoption

Boris Gindis

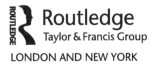

Routledge
Taylor & Francis Group

LONDON AND NEW YORK

First published 2019 by Routledge

2 Park Square, Milton Park, Abingdon, Oxon, OX14 4RN
605 Third Avenue, New York, NY 10017

Routledge is an imprint of the Taylor & Francis Group, an informa business

First issued in paperback 2020

Library of Congress Cataloguing in Publication Data
A catalog record for this book has been requested

ISBN: 978-1-138-57203-4 (hbk)
ISBN: 978-0-367-72833-5 (pbk)

Typeset in Sabon
by Apex CoVantage, LLC

To Tatyana: Your support and care made this book possible; indeed, when you read these lines, they are the only new ones for you in the book—all the rest was the outcome of our joint/shared efforts.

Contents

Tables

Acknowledgments

This book has three sources, three pillars, so to speak: clinical experience, research/reading, and communication with colleagues and adoptive parents. These contacts, interactions, and consultations should be specially recognized.

My great thanks and gratitude to the staff and consultants at the BGCenter, particularly to Ida Jeltova, Chun Dong, Carol Napier, Elkhonon Goldberg, Marina Muchnick, Marie Pruden, and Shylamit Ryshick; to my friends, co-authors, and colleagues Marie Pruden, Carol Lidz, Alex Kozulin, and Patty Cogan; to Dmitry Zlotsky, who influenced my writing style; to a group of adoptive parents at Families for Russian and Ukrainian Adoption, Eastern Europe Adoption Coalition, Families with Children From China, and Latin America Parents Association in particular. These individuals and groups have served as inspiration and as sounding boards for my thoughts and actions over the last thirty years. And last, but surely not least, is my family: my wife, Tatyana, who helps me in all possible ways, and my son, Elliot, whose books served me as stimulation and encouragement.

Introduction

The "Unnatural" Natural Experiment

Our perception is determined by habits, preferences, and social stereotypes that are far from being universal. But there is at least one exception: a child. A tiny human always draws warm feelings. Every baby is created to be irresistible: it is the ticket to the infant's survival. Whether its helplessness or purity, when meeting those large or slanted, brown, blue, or black eyes, we can't resist compassion. It seems like imagination is the only force that can break that mold of enchantment. Let's use it to run one mental experiment.

Imagine a scientist, unlike any who exists in the world. An evil scientist who shares none of our empathy and who decided to study the tolerance of a human cub—in a mind game everything is possible. The scientist has control over things we can't even dream about in real life. His tools are misfortunes; his methods are wicked. Immoral but meticulous, the evil scientist (ES) begins his experiments long before birth. His choice for a mother goes to the least suitable candidate. Ill-fed and homeless, she smokes and drinks. She is a drug addict and a prostitute, unfamiliar with or unwilling to follow the very basic precautions for expecting mothers. Using our imagination for his vile purposes, ES triggers the birth to happen well before its time. The baby appears to the world prematurely and undernourished.

Had the experiment ended here, the doctors would rush to the delivery ward, place the baby under a heat lamp, and hook the baby to the sensors and vitamin-rich IVs. But ES isn't done yet. He makes his experimental child suffer from hunger and cold. Nobody responds to the baby's cry; nobody feeds it on time; nobody keeps it warm. The mother neglects the duties imprinted in all the mothers in the world. She leaves the child unattended and hungry more and more often, and, finally, she disappears for good.

Without help, the baby is doomed, but death plays no part in the ES's research. Introducing a social component to his tests, the ES commits the child to a state-run institution—an orphanage. Understaffed and overworked, the adults there barely have time to take care of the kids' basic needs. They come and go. Their frequent rotation makes no attachment possible. To get even the minimum amount of affection, the unfortunates must elbow their way for attention.

And yet, despite the ordeal, as if determined to prove the ES wrong, the child does the impossible. He adapts to the inhospitable world and clings to life like ivy to a rock. With flexibility and resilience, the little *Homo sapiens* learns survival tricks and finds ways to avoid pain.

That's when ES plays his last trick and brings a couple of strangers into the child's life. They look unlike everybody else he knows. Their smile is confusing. They speak a strange language. They take the child to a country where nothing works the way it's supposed to. The food, the clothes, and the manners are disorienting. All ties to the past are severed. The only language the child understands is useless. The child now must learn the new language and adjust to a new life. Having been disadvantaged all his life, he must now compete with children who have been fortunate to escape the attention of ES. The horrors of his previous life pursue the child and mold his perception of the world and his relationships with new surroundings. Finally, the mind game, or rather the nightmare, is over.

In real life, no scientific committee would ever approve such an experiment, and a grant application for such a study would be rejected on the grounds of cruelty. Our humane society condemns the very premise of such research.

And yet this project is well under way. The name of this natural experiment is "international adoption." It's a widespread phenomenon. During the last 30 years, North America (USA and Canada) accepted near half a million children who come from all over the world: Eastern Europe, China, Latin America, Southeast Asia, and Africa. The experiment described earlier as unthinkable is more real than one would want to believe. It is happening right now, and every day children with the history presented earlier enter our society.

Why This Book Was Written, and What This Book Is All About

In the murky January morning of 1989, I was sitting in my office in a small private clinic in New York. "An unusual patient is scheduled for today," the secretary said. In the waiting room, I saw a middle-aged, elegantly dressed woman with a tiny pale boy who appeared to be about 6 or 7 years old.

At that time, and in that clinic, I worked mostly with bilingual (Russian-speaking) patients, and although the woman had a typical American last name, I greeted her in Russian.

"Sorry, doctor," she said. "I do not speak Russian."

I apologized and switched to English.

The woman handed me a folder and said, "This is my son Misha, and here are his medical records, all in Russian."

I greeted the boy in English and extended my hand to him. He was visibly scared and clung to his mother.

"Sorry, doctor." The woman smiled. "My son does not speak English, only Russian."

"How come?" I asked, puzzled. "You said he is your son. You speak only English, and he understands only Russian?"

The mother replied, "He is only seven days in the US. We adopted him from an orphanage in Moscow, Russia."

This was the first time I heard the words "international adoption" and met my first patient, a former orphan from Russia.

Very soon, international adoptees constituted the majority of my patients. I found myself being deeply emotionally involved in the international adoption endeavor. I made personal friends and met esteemed colleagues in this field. I witnessed the entire spectrum of human emotions of extreme intensity, encountered mostly challenging and fascinating psychological assignments, and, finally, I have been living through the rather rare experience of actually affecting human lives for the better.

The book that you have in your hands is not a memoir by any stretch of the imagination: this is a research endeavor. But I cannot dissociate myself from what is a rich, exhilarating venture for the last 30 years of my life, and you will see rather emotional overtones in my research discourse.

In 1992, I organized the Center for Cognitive-Developmental Assessment and Remediation (known for its shorter name, BGCenter[1]), which specializes in working with internationally adopted, post-institutionalized children. With other colleagues, native speakers of Chinese and Spanish, and, occasionally, using translators from other languages, we did initial assessments and screenings in native languages of children adopted literally from the entire world, from Eastern Europe to Latin America, from China to Ethiopia.

As time progressed, there were reevaluations of my former patients, so I have accumulated a variety of longitudinal data, seeing the same patients sometimes from two to six (sic!) times during the first post-adoption decade. The data would also come from parents, other professionals, and participants of conferences and workshops. Through all these channels of communication and interaction, I remained bewildered with the commonality of psychological problems of international adoptees at different stages of their development. Despite unique individual traits, various racial backgrounds, and cultural differences, they share many key features.

Starting from abandonment and institutionalization, every one of these children, without exception, has gone through painful experiences that follow them through their formative years; distress and misery impede their development, which is further hindered by the very process of international adoption. Instead of solving all problems, the arrival in the new motherland introduces new challenges. Familial life with its relationships was an unchartered terrain for the majority of international adoptees. Their orphanage survival skills turned out to be useless and even destructive for them. English was a shock. The native language that used to be at the core of social liaisons becomes a burden, and the majority will discard their first language abruptly. The loss of culture is just as imminent for "older" adoptees. And, finally, even for those adopted as infants or toddlers, the American educational system presented a challenge for many more years.

I felt that there was something that produced similar disabilities, calamities, and delays. I was looking for the explanatory principle that would organize and make my empirical knowledge a legitimate part of a high-level conceptualization. In my search, I turned to what is known as chronic post-traumatic stress, which could be blamed for international adoptees' social, school, and family problems. I studied the post-traumatic stress disorder (PTSD) research literature and soon came to the conclusion that it is too narrow an explanation, not covering an array of symptoms I observed in my patients. After all, PTSD originates in a discrete, traumatic incident rather than an ongoing pattern of repetitive traumatization. PTSD means a specific response to stimuli that are reminders of the traumatic incidents (so-called triggers) and has a set of well-defined symptoms. There was no question that some of my patients had a clear-cut PTSD condition, but they have other conditions as well that were developmental in nature. In clinical practice, when PTSD can't account for all the symptoms present, other diagnoses are often used to explain additional symptoms. I feel like the part is mistaken for the whole, and the overall picture is clouded by this PTSD symptomatology. I observed in a majority of my patients that development was mediated by a powerful factor that still is to be defined, analyzed, and addressed by different means of remediation.

Slowly but surely, complex childhood trauma emerged as the basic explanatory concept. The most helpful were publications of B. A. van der Kolk., A. Schore, P. Ogden, and their associates that emerged in the late '90s and resulted in the formulation of the most heuristic notion of developmental trauma disorder. Indeed, the most damaging for my patients was neglect and its extreme form of total abandonment. This tragic action damages the very core of human nature—social connectedness—and in the evolutionary course means the annihilation of a human being. Further, my patients were living through repetitive and pervasive highly stressful events and conditions, mostly within the interpersonal context, which resulted in the wide-ranging and long-lasting adverse impact on the development and maturation of their high psychological functions. I finally realized that complex childhood trauma mediates the overall development in a very profound way: many enigmas of development in my patients were explained, and the traditional remedial methodology gave way to the system of scaffolding and compensation.

Traditionally, complex childhood trauma is studied in the same cultural and linguistic environment. This book offers a new perspective on development mediated by trauma, when a radical change in the social situation of development has occurred: from institutional care to family life, from extreme deprivation and neglect to attentive and protective middle-class style of parenting, from native language and culture to sweeping changes in the cultural/linguistic setting. To the best of my knowledge, there is no research on the trauma that occurs when a traumatized person completely changes his or her social situation of development.

This entire book has to be viewed as the search for the answer to the essence of complex childhood trauma and how it mediates the development of a child from birth to young adulthood. In this book, internationally adopted, post-institutionalized children are presented as an extreme case of developmental trauma disorder, which makes clear that some very essential characteristics of this condition may be extrapolated to a wider populace of children who are victims of complex childhood trauma. Within the last 30 years, the "big picture" of international adoption emerged. Although there is not much of a "rosy" color in this picture, the fact of life is that the majority of international adoptees are able to overcome, to different degrees, the consequences of early and prolong traumatization and join the general population as productive, self-sufficient, and law-abiding members of society. This is the proof of human resilience and resourcefulness, and a testimony of our society's ability to provide sufficient support and guidance for reaching this status by international adoptees. If this book will contribute to the "know-how" to help current and future international adoptees, I would consider my mission successfully accomplished.

Note

1. www.bgcenter.com

1 Contemporary International Adoption—A Unique Social/Cultural Phenomenon

An Introduction to International Adoption

History: International adoption is not a modern invention. The biblical Book of Exodus described the first "documented" case when, fearing for her baby's life after the Pharaoh's decree to drown all newborn Hebrew boys, a Jewish mother placed her son in a wicker basket and let the waters of the Nile River carry it downstream. Luckily, the Pharaoh's daughter, while resting on the shore, discovered the makeshift raft stuck amid reeds and bulrushes. The boy was so beautiful that she took him to the palace, adopted him, and named him Moses.

Fast-forward a few thousand years and miles. On a relatively small scale, international adoption has been in existence in North America and Western Europe throughout history with noticeable surges after World War II and the wars in Korea and Vietnam (Johnston, 2017). The famous pre-World War II *Kindertransport* of more than 10,000 mostly Jewish children from Nazi Germany to England, the adoption of Holocaust survivors in Israel and Western Europe, and Vietnamese "boat people" parentless children adoptions in the US in the early 1970s were all modern episodes of international adoption on a somewhat smaller scale.

And then something occurred that had never happened in human history in such a short period of time and on a such vast scale: the last 30 years (1987–2017) witnessed a sharp spike in adoption numbers, resulting in almost a million and a half children adopted by industrialized countries of North America, Australia, and Western Europe (Jones & Placek, 2017).

Thus, according to the Bureau of Consular Affairs, US Department of State statistics,[1] 395,324 internationally adopted children entered the US from 1987 to 2017, with the numbers peaking in 2004–2006 and gradually declining, particularly after 2013. Indeed, never before in human history were so many children from so many countries and for such a short period of time adopted by a single country. The dynamic of international adoption within the last 25 years is seen in Table 1.1:

Table 1.1 US International Adoptions by Regions/Countries 1990 Through 2016

From: Johnston, R. (2017) Historical international adoption statistics, US and world, last updated April 2017 and available at www.johnstonsarchive.net/policy/adoptionstatsintl.html

Geography

According to the report of the UN Department of Economic and Social Affairs "Child Adoption: Trends and Policies" (2009, p. XV), the main countries receiving foreign children were (in descending order): the US, Spain, France, Italy, Canada, Sweden, Germany, Australia and New Zealand (together), Switzerland, and the Netherlands. Until 2008, the US maintained its leading position, adopting more children than all other receiving countries combined (Selman, 2012). Since 2009, Europe has accepted more than 50% of all internationally adopted children. According to statistics from the US Department of State Bureau of Consular Affairs,[2] over half of the children adopted internationally in the US arrived from China and countries in Eastern Europe (mostly from countries of the former Soviet Union). In Southeast Asia, South Korea and Vietnam are the leading donors. In Latin America, Guatemala and Columbia contributed the majority of all adoptees. Africa concluded the list with the bulk of adoptees coming mostly from Ethiopia.

Gender

Consistently in each year since 1987, the adoption of females has prevailed: girls have made up about 62% of all international adoptees (Selman, 2012).

Age of Adoption

This is an important statistical indicator for the understanding of research data in general and the content of this book in particular. Initially, from late 1980 to the first decade of the 21st century, the vast majority (almost 80%) of internationally adopted children were infants and toddlers between the ages 3 months to 3 years. Slowly but steadily, the percentage of older (ages 5 to 12 and above) adoptees grew: if in 1999 the fraction of those international adoptees who were older than 5 was 13%, in 2011, the proportion had risen to 28% and keeps growing (US Department of State, n.d.).

What is worth noticing is that most of the research on international adoption published between 1990 and 2013 was done on children adopted before their second to fourth birthdays, with very little research on the so-called older adoptees, adopted after the age of 5. In practically all longitudinal studies, the subjects were initially infants and toddlers who spent the first 6 to 36 months in an institution. Exceptionally rare investigators have dealt with adopted preadolescents and adolescents despite that each year since 2010, "older adoptees," ages 5 to 17, have constituted almost a quarter of all internationally adopted children, and this is definitely a growing tendency.

International Adoption as a Controversial Subject

Similar to every high-profile human undertaking, especially one that involves large monetary transactions, international adoption is not immune to controversy and has its passionate proponents and ardent adversaries.

Controversy Among General Public

There are many reasons for the upsurge of international adoption in the affluent Western societies, such as an inability to have a biological child (50%), desire to expand the family (68%), and willingness to give a child a permanent home (81%) (Ela, 2011). According to the 2007 National Survey of Adoptive Parents[3], adoptive parents were pursuing an international adoption because they thought adoption from the US would be too difficult (65%), wanted an infant (63%), and wanted a closed adoption (no contact between birth and adoptive families) (51%). For a more detailed discussion, please see *Adoption Nation* by A. Pertman (2011). I can add to Pertman's analysis one observation of my own: the expansion of the Internet and international adoption coincide in time, and I firmly believe that the Internet has fueled international adoption tremendously.

As an idea, international adoption is a most dignified one. It favors both sides: the parents who have emotional desire (love) and material resources to share and a child who needs the first as well as the second.

In general, international adoption provides an existential benefit for both children and parents. Adopted children of all ages are better off than their peers who remain in orphanages. A lot of adopted children, initially significantly delayed, were able to catch up to their age group in physical health, cognitive functioning, academic performance, and adaptive behavior (Van IJzendoorn & Juffer, 2006; Van IJzendoorn, Bakermans-Kranenburg, & Juffer, 2007; Vandivere, Malm, & Radel, 2009). Overall, the majority of parents who adopted internationally were satisfied with their decision and their relationship with adopted children (Clark, Thigpen, & Moeller-Yates, 2006; Ji, Brooks, Barth, & Kim, 2010; Whitten & Weaver, 2010).

Still, as with any human creation, adoption has its pitfalls. The Schuster Institute for Investigative Journalism[4] cites numerous cases of fraud and corruption in the practice of international adoption (Graff, 2009, 2010a, 2010b). The gap between supply and demand creates opportunities for abusing an endeavor, however noble it is at its core. The frequent cases of corruption forced some countries to curtail their supply of children. The United Nations organization was not going to tolerate widespread mistreatment of children, and an international agreement known as the Hague Convention on the Protection of Children and Co-operation in Respect of Intercountry Adoption (known as the "Hague Adoption Convention") was created to establish safeguards and ensure that intercountry adoptions take place in the best interests of children[5].

But even when no laws are broken, some opponents view the loss of language, culture, and identity as a major drawback of international adoptions. Quoting Pauline Turner-Strong, an American anthropologist who researched intercultural adoption (2001, p. 468), "*adoption across political and cultural borders may simultaneously be an act of violence and an act of love, an excruciating rupture and a generous incorporation, an appropriation of valued resources and a constitution of personal ties.*"

Controversy Among Research Community

I have been following the research studies on international adoption in the US, Canada, Australia, and Western Europe since the beginning of the 1990s and cannot free myself from conflicting and confusing impressions. In a way, the situation resembles the old Indian tale about seven blind people describing an elephant after touching different parts of the animal. Too many publications had been using nonrepresentative adoption samples, questionable methodology and means of investigations (mostly questionnaires of adoptive parents and behavior scales standardized on middle-class Western population), and reported outcomes that hardly can be generalized for the other groups of international adoptees. With many thousands of children adopted from the third world within the last 30 years, the study of this extremely heterogenous cohort produces findings that are at times inconsistent at best and contradictory at worst. For example, there is a group of publications that described a generally positive outcome of international adoption for mental health and achievements of international adoptees (Ijzendoorn & Juffer, 2005a, 2006; Wright & Flynn, 2006; Bakermans-Kranenburg, Van IJzendoorn, & Juffer, 2008; Van den Dries, Juffer, Van IJzendoorn, & Bakermans-Kranenburg, 2009; Compton, 2016). Still, no less authoritative publications suggested that substantial numbers of internationally adopted children, as they grew up in new motherlands, became maladjusted, with higher than average rates of educational and mental health problems (Hjern, Lindblad, & Vinnerljung, 2002; van Ijzendoorn & Juffer, 2005b; Ford, Vostanis, Meltzer, & Goodman, 2007; Beckett, Castle, Rutter, & Sonuga-Barke, 2010; Juffer et al., 2012). This is not surprising given the marked variations in orphanages, measurement instruments, duration of exposure to the institutional life, ages at adoption and ages of assessment among other relevant parameters.

Our initial knowledge of contemporary international adoptees originated from two relatively small samples of Romanian children adopted in Canada and in Great Britain between 1887 and 1991. Pioneering works of two groups of research under the leadership of E. Ames (Canada) and M. Rutter (England) provided substantial initial data, including valuable longitudinal reports. However, this cohort of Romanian orphans, mostly infants and toddlers, arrived from the most inhumane environment, being extremely deprived, neglected, and likely neurologically damaged. To consider them as a representative group of all international adoptees would be erroneous. Furthermore, we know relatively little about the post-adoption outcomes for children being adopted after the age of 5 years, and this category includes every fourth child adopted internationally.

Internationally adopted post-institutionalized children, as a group, have a specific set of characteristics that distinguishes them from domestic adoptees, from the offspring of recently immigrated families, and from children in need of special education. Our attempts to apply insights and experiences with domestically adopted children or with the youngsters from recently immigrated families may not be helpful in relation to internationally adopted orphans. Parents, educators, and professionals alike have been facing a new frontier, navigating uncharted waters, so to speak. Our knowledge about international adoptees as a group is still fragmentary, but one assumption seems to be correct: their adjustment to life in a family versus life in an institution, to a new physical and technological environment, to a new cultural and social milieu, and to a new school setting is determined by many developmental and individual differences, with internalized trauma being the most prominent.

Changing Landscape of International Adoption

One glance at Table 1.1 (Johnston, 2017) shows a fourfold reduction in the number of entry visas for international adoptees issued by the US in 2016 in comparison with 2004 (22,989 entry visas versus 5,372, respectively). The number of intercountry adoptions to the top-14 receiving countries worldwide for the same time period fell at an even faster rate, as evident from the Annual Report on Intercountry Adoptions[6].

Along with the reduction in numbers, we see the changes in the racial component. The proportion of adopted children being raised by parents of a different race or ethnic group rose by 50% between 1999 and 2016 (Zill, 2017a). While international adoptions are not necessarily or intentionally interracial, they often turn out that way when white American and European couples adopt children from China, Guatemala, or Ethiopia.

Countries that have served as major sources of adoptable infants are undergoing changes in their adoption policies. Russia banned foreign adoptions to parents from the US and some other countries in 2013. International agreements aimed at reducing corruption and exploitation of impoverished families are having unintended consequences, such as cutting off adoptions from some countries, expanding paperwork, delays, bureaucratic hurdles that prospective parents must overcome, and raising the age of adopted children (Selman, 2009; Compton, 2016).

As of now, we see two distinct trends in the field of international adoption that will likely be noticeable in the future. First, fewer countries will be on the "donating" side and, due to changing policies in these countries, special needs and older children may constitute the largest percentage of children available for international adoption. Second, due to improved pre-adoption care (e.g., better conditions in orphanages worldwide) and greater availability of post-adoption services in receiving countries, adopted children will have better prospects for development than in the past.

International adoption is alive and active, but it changes its qualitative and quantitative characteristics. As presented in Pinderhughes, Matthews, Georgia Deoudes, and Pertman (2013, p. 12),

> *Intercountry adoption has changed comprehensively and is still in the midst of its transformation from a robust but largely unmonitored process through which tens of thousands of infants and toddlers moved into new homes annually, into a smaller but better-regulated system serving primarily children who are older and/or have special needs.*

Internationally Adopted, Post-Institutionalized (IAPI) Children—Definition and Specificity

For the sake of simplicity, I refer to internationally adopted, post-institutionalized orphans as "IAPI children" or as "international adoptees" or "internationally adopted children" with the understanding that these children:

- are born outside of the North America and Western Europe in different racial groups with various languages and diverse social/cultural environments, but mostly in the countries of the third world;
- are legal orphans, as defined by US Immigration Law: "A child may be considered an orphan because of the death or disappearance of, abandonment or desertion by, or separation or loss from, both parents. The child of an unwed mother or surviving parent may be considered an orphan if that parent is unable to care for the child properly and has, in writing, irrevocably released the child for emigration and adoption"[7];
- subsequently resided in nonfamily settings, such as orphanages, hospitals, or foster care;
- have been legally adopted by citizens of economically advanced countries and brought to these countries to live permanently with their new families. Adoption is the legal process that establishes a parent-child relationship between individuals who are not related biologically[8];
- are ages 3 months through 17 years at the time of adoption.

In fact, the IAPI contingent is consists of three groups: "true orphans" who do not have living parents; "social orphans" who have at least one living parent, who, for a variety of reasons, is unable, unwilling, or unfit to rear the child; and "refused orphans"—those abandoned soon after birth with no information about biological parents (most adoptees from China and many from Russia).

Despite their unique physical traits, age, various backgrounds, and distinct language and cultural differences, nearly all international adoptees display the prominent common features.

First, every one of the international adoptees had to go through painful, trauma-producing experiences in their pre-adoptive lives. Like in the thought experiment of the evil scientist, traumas follow these children throughout their formative years; distress and misery impede their development, which is further hindered by the very process of international adoption. In addition to a prolonged and severe trauma, prospective international adoptees often have genetic and epigenetic-based problems passed to them by their stressed out and deranged biological parents; they often have an upset microbiome due to environmental toxins and deprivations before adoption. After adoption, they routinely suffer from the socially induced trauma of not being able to fit in because of the differences in cultural background, lack of language mastery, and overall accumulated delays.

As much as the prospective parents want to believe in the abundance of healthy babies in the third world "donor" countries, this is no more than a myth. The majority of children available for adoption, one way or another, were affected by their physical and social environments and can be deeply traumatized, physically handicapped, and neurologically impaired. As aptly formulated in the Evan B. Donaldson Institute report (2010)[9] page 1,

> *Most adopted children, because they suffered early deprivation or maltreatment, come to their new families with elevated risks for developmental, physical, psychological, emotional, or behavioral challenges. Among the factors linked with these higher risks are the following: prenatal malnutrition and low birth weight, prenatal exposure to toxic substances, older age at adoption, early deprivation, abuse or neglect, multiple placements, and emotional conflicts related to loss and identity issues.*

The troubles of IAPI children can be summarized as follows:

- Medical issues: problems that have developmental impact—e.g., premature birth, low birth weight, severe malnutrition during the infant years, prenatal exposure to alcohol and drugs, neurological impairments of different origins.
- Social and educational issues: educational neglect and cultural deprivation during pre-adoption years, poor language development and abrupt first-language attrition after adoption, inappropriate school placement, and lack of remediation after adoption.
- Mental health issues: developmental trauma disorder and/or chronic PTSD as a result of repeated traumatization, institutionally shaped personality, and predisposition to attachment difficulties. Possible continuation of a chain of traumatic experiences after adoption: mismatched family, traumatic school experiences, rejection by peers.

Second, the language of the accepting country becomes adoptees' native language with their first languages being subjected to rapid attrition. The majority of IAPI children start learning their new language—whether English, French, Italian, or Dutch, etc.—several years later than their peers, and their way of acquisition of the new language is different from the "typical" ways of mastering language in their peers.

Third, contrary to popular belief, rather than solving all problems, the child's arrival in the new motherland introduces new challenges in addition to the old ones. Family life with its relationships is unchartered territory for children used to orphanages. In the new circumstances, none of their proven behavioral models apply. They go through the painful process of discarding their native language and learning new language as a survival skill. The loss of culture for an "older" adoptee is just as imminent. And, finally, even for those adopted as infants or toddlers, the Western educational system often presents a painful challenge for years to come.

What are the differences between children from the domestic foster care population in the US in comparison with IAPI children? Domestically adopted children are the US-born infants placed with an adoptive family by their birth parents who legally consent to this. Domestically adopted children are typically infants, often adopted immediately after birth, while the IAPI children range from toddlers to teenagers. The availability of the medical and social history of the child and his or her birth parents is incomparable between international and domestic adoption. In domestic adoption, the prospective adoptive parents can examine the birth and health circumstances of the child they are accepting. For example, if the family is not comfortable adopting a child who may have been exposed to alcohol in utero, this family will not be considered for such a situation. This is not the case in international adoption. Finally, another difference is that English is a native language for domestically adopted children, and a whole range of problems related to first-language attrition and learning new language does not exist for them. Typically, there are no drastic cultural differences between adoptive families and children in domestic foster care, even if they are from different social stratum.

A Trip From Point A (Orphanage) to Point B (Adoptive Family)

The IAPI children have to live through a mind-boggling, rapid change of their social situation of development: literally in one night, a child transfers from an institution to a family life, from an objectively neglected, traumatic, and impoverished environment to an objectively enriched, safe, and optimal for normal development setting. (The subjective perception of these changes is a different matter, however.) In the new and objectively favorable developmental milieu, traumatic experiences may continue as the previous trauma mediates the transfer and related adjustment. Both research and clinical practice show that too many IAPI children experience difficulty in learning, forming social bonds, and functioning age appropriately in major domains of life. To understand the psychological essence of this phenomenon, we need to consider both points of this incredible passage—from point A (orphanage) to point B (adoptive family).

Orphanage as Social Institution: A Case of Structural Neglect

Orphanages exist in many countries as a major means of addressing the issue of parentless children. In the general public perception in North America and Western Europe, the word "orphanage" has a negative connotation, mostly associated with Charles Dickens's *Oliver Twist* novel and the recent horror of Romanian warehouses for unwanted children. According to Goodwin (1994, p. 416), former New York City Mayor Fiorello H. La Guardia once exclaimed, "*The worst mother is better than the best orphanage.*" In 2017, J. K. Rowling, the author of the Harry Potter series, wrote in one of her tweets[10], "*Orphanages cause irreparable damage, even those that are well run.*" Photos and documentaries about the misery of neglected children in Romanian orphanages of the early 1990s are still in the public consciousness (see *Growing Up in a Romanian Orphanage*, BBC News, 2016[11]).

Typical orphanages as a means of addressing the issue of parentless children do not exist in North America: the last such institution for orphans was closed in the US in 1979 (Keiger, 1996). In their place, there are modern boarding schools, residential treatment centers, and group homes, though foster care remains the most common form of support for children who are waiting for adoption. In general, the system of foster care is the most common "family-like" substitution for orphanages in the developed countries of the West.

I dare to disagree with Mr. La Guardia's emotional statement that "the worst mother is better than the best orphanage." The reader should realize that the majority of children accepted to orphanages all over the world come from environments that typically are much worse than an orphanage. As an example, let us take the Russian Federation, which was the second donating country after China in international adoption worldwide (from 1989 through 2013).

According to the official Russian accounts, up to 95% (data for the year 2013) of children in the orphanages are "social orphans" (at least one of the parents is alive) coming from the lowest socioeconomic strata of the society (Valeeva & Kalimulin, 2015). The reasons for accepting children into a state-run institution in the status of "social orphan" are the following:

Rejection of a newborn child in maternity ward; forced removal of children from their families because of parental rights deprivation on the basis of parents' alcoholism, drug addiction, child abuse, asocial way of life, incarceration of a parent for a serious crime, parent's permanent mental health disorders, incapacitating physical disability.

(Valeeva & Kalimulin, 2015, p. 212)

In the legal documentation of adoption from Russia, Kazakhstan, Ukraine, and other countries of the former Soviet Union, there are descriptions of neglect and abuse in biological families that are beyond the imagination of a Western reader. No prenatal care was reported for practically all children admitted to the orphanage as "social orphans." When the state takes these children away from their "caregivers" (the word "mother" is not appropriate here), the children are sick, malnourished, delayed, and terrified (Dubrovina, 1991; Johnson, 2000; Gindis, 2005; the St. Petersburg—USA Orphanage Research Team, 2009). Practically all were initially placed in the so-called quarantine (an isolated infectious-disease ward) for a month to check if they have contagious diseases. Only after this procedure were children placed into an orphanage according to their ages: those younger than 3 were placed into a "Baby House," those between 3 and 7 into a "Children's Home," and those of school age into the so-called school-internat, an orphanage with a school on premises or in the neighborhood (Gindis, 2005; Shipitsyna, 2008). In the vast majority of cases, placement in an orphanage objectively changes the social situation of development for the better: new admittances get relatively normal and regular nutrition, proper (even by Western standards) medical care, and a relatively safe environment (Gindis, 2005; Shipitsyna, 2008; The St. Petersburg—USA Orphanage Research Team, 2009). In Russia, some of these children are placed in the so-called corrective (or "specialized") orphanages for children with physical disabilities, neurological weaknesses, developmental delays, and cognitive limitations. These orphanages are under the auspice of the Ministry of Health, not the Ministry of Education, as regular orphanages are. Those "specialized" orphanages receive more financial support from the state in comparison with regular orphanages (Dubrovina, 1991; Shipitsyna, 2008). The staff is more stable, and nutrition and medical care are better than in the regular orphanages as reported by the St. Petersburg—USA Orphanage Research Team (2009). According to statistics, near half of all children adopted before their third birthday in North America and Western Europe came from the specialized Baby Houses (Johnson, 2000; Miller, 2005).

Does an orphanage, as an institution, inherently and automatically produce adverse childhood experience? The answer to this question is not as evident as it may appear. Thus, there are positive views on the orphanage as an establishment (McCall, 1998) presented in the book *Rethinking Orphanages for the 21st Century*. The book gives a compelling case that unwanted children are cared for much better in the private-sector orphanages run by churches or other charitable organizations than in the existing foster care system. The authors remind us that worldwide there are many thousands of parentless children who remain on the streets or in refugee camps, for whom an orphanage would be a desirable alternative.

On the other hand, the current outlook on orphanages as an "inherently" traumatic institutional experience remains unchanged: the general conclusion of more than 30 years of investigation on the outcomes of institutional rearing is that former orphanage residents are well behind their family-raised peers in physical and mental health, cognitive/academic functioning, and social/emotional adjustment. Studies of children who were warehoused in large orphanages in Romania with only minimal care and social interactions have found that early institutionalization, characterized by extreme sensory, cognitive, linguistic, and psychosocial deprivation have a profoundly negative impact on development: adverse childhood experiences of the early institutionalization are "biologically embedded," changing the structure and function of the brain, and modifying the foundation for future development.

Scientific analysis of the orphanage as an institution would be very helpful in understanding this issue. However, this is hardly possible due to the extreme heterogeneity of such institutions, even within one country, not to mention the differences among orphanages in various countries. Nevertheless, Gunnar (2001), using such a vague discriminator as "the quality of care," attempted to hypothetically categorize existing orphanages into three groups:

1. Institutions characterized by global deprivation of the child's health, nutrition, stimulation, and relationship needs;
2. Institutions with adequate health and nutrition support, but deprivation of the child's stimulation and relationship needs;
3. Institutions that meet all needs except for stable, long-term relationships with consistent caregivers.

Accepting this classification, a group of researches (Van IJzendoorn et al., 2011) suggested that basically all, even the best orphanages,

> *inevitably deprive children of sensitive reciprocal interactions with stable caregivers. In this respect, many if not most institutions are characterized by structural neglect, which may include minimum physical resources, unfavorable staffing patterns, and socially-emotionally inadequate caregiver-child interactions. Structural neglect should be considered a special case of child maltreatment.*
>
> (p. 11)

The authors continued,

> *Structural neglect is probably the main and most widespread form of institutional maltreatment, pointing to the fact that, by their arrangement and form of operation, institutions fail to respond to children's basic needs for stable and positive personal relationships as well as for adequate care and stimulation.*
>
> (p. 17)

Accepting "structural neglect" as the main negative characteristic of an institution, we still have to realize that for the majority of orphanage residents, the institutional experience contributes substantially to their concurrent and persistent developmental deficiencies caused by initial pre-orphanage traumatization, genetic inheritance, pre-birth exposure to different teratogens, and other adverse factors. In other words, developmental calamities of IAPI children cannot be attributed to institutional rearing alone: genetics, prenatal conditions (e.g., maternal exposure to drugs, alcohol, and other teratogens), birth complications (e.g., low birth weight, hypoxia, poor Apgar scores), and pre-orphanage experience (e.g., life in a dysfunctional, abusive and neglectful family) all have the potential to produce or significantly facilitate the negative developmental outcomes.

In contemporary research literature, the most prominent evidences that institutional "structural neglect" interposes significant impact are as follows:

1. The delayed development of institutionalized children and their catchup growth (in different degrees in different domains) after adoption—all these in spite of variations in institutions and families (MacLean, 2003; Juffer & Van IJzendoorn, 2005a; Juffer et al., 2012).
2. A "dose-response" effect that is observed in many survivors of institutional care: the longer time in an institution means deeper developmental impairments. However, the relation between time in the orphanage and the negative consequences is not clear, and, as stated by some researches, may not be linear (Morison & Ellwood, 2000; Juffer et al., 2012; Gunnar, 2001; MacLean, 2003; Rutter, Kreppner, & O'Connor, 2001; Rutter et al., 2010).
3. Intervention studies, demonstrating improvement in children's development when the institutional environment is improved, in particular the social aspect of child rearing (the St. Petersburg—USA Orphanage Research Team, 2009; Bakermans-Kranenburg et al., 2008).

What appears as a verified fact is that, consistent with a "cumulative risk theory" (Rutter, 1999), the institution may have provided an environment that not only failed to remediate the existing problems but also may have exacerbated previous difficulties and created additional ones.

Although it is common knowledge now that children reared in institutions are at greater risk for atypical development, we do not possess yet a specific knowledge of how different types of neglect and deprivation impact the neurobehavioral development of young children of different ages against the background of a specific child's genetic makeup and prenatal conditions.

Further, discussing institutions (orphanages, transitional group foster care, hospitals, etc.) as the cause of problems, we cannot ignore one obvious fact: the different developmental outcomes of being institutionalized. In other words, there are significant individual differences in children exposed to the same life in an orphanage. While some children suffered extreme damage, others who lived in the same orphanage for the same period of time could demonstrate adaptive behavior close to age expectations, be receptive to remediation, and, finally, could successfully mix with a crowd of their peers in the general population after adoption. Why does this happen? Is it possible to distinguish a specific feature in the orphanage environment that causes the most damage? Or, as noted by Van IJzendoorn et al. (2011), are all characteristics of an orphanage *"performed in a concert, facilitating and reinforcing each other—the synergetic effect of life in institution is greater than each afflicting factor alone"*? (p. 18).

The fact of life, observed in my clinical practice on many occasions, is that some children remain resilient even in the most adverse settings. A study of the nature and mechanisms of their resilience from many perspectives (from epigenetic to higher forms of socialization) may give us answers to many questions about rearing parentless children. Still, I fully agree with my colleagues cited earlier (see also.: Van den Dries, Juffer, Van IJzendoorn, & Bakermans-Kranenburg, 2009) that the quality of interpersonal relationships in an orphanage is the most powerful factor (above the quality of food, shelter, and medical support) in prevention of many institutional calamities.

Clinical Case: Alex—An Enigmatic Source of Strength

I completed the initial screening of Alex upon his arrival: I saw a physically fragile 7-year-old boy, the son of a Russian mother and Estonian father who had lived in an Estonian orphanage for as long as he remembered and had the usual history of abandonment, abuse, and neglect. In his medical pre-adoption documentation, I saw a "laundry list" of different maladies, though none of them were significant. My recommendations included regular education placement with some supportive services. However, Alex never received any therapies or remedial education in US schools.

Alex was adopted by a couple from upstate New York. Four years later, his adoptive mother died from cancer. His father, a retired Navy officer, himself with poor health conditions, called my office regularly, and we talked about Alex and his progress. I saw Alex in my office one more time when he was about 15, due to his father's request, who believed that the boy was depressed. I assured the father that Alex was emotionally stable and a fully functional, successful adolescent, and his sad appearance was just what it was—a façade. I spoke to his math teacher, who became close to the boy during his high school years. The teacher characterized Alex as a "wonderful young man, somewhat reserved, shy and rarely smiling, but highly self-disciplined and goal-oriented. He is a hard worker with a knack for exact sciences, the best president of our school math club I ever had." Alex turned out to be a good athlete as well, particularly in cross-country skiing. As his father said, the boy practically ran the house, doing food shopping, cleaning, and taking care of his father's chronic illness.

When Alex was 16, the local police awarded him with an honor plaque for helping to save two little girls who fell through the ice at a nearby lake. Two years later, having received a recommendation from his state senator, Alex applied for the military academy and was accepted. His father sent me the pictures taken during four years of military training and finally at the graduation ceremony. At the age of 23, Alex emerged as a mature, accomplished young man, whom our society and his father could be proud of.

Fighting the lot cast to him by fate, this boy showed tremendous resilience. He managed to overcome his past and tough post-adoption conditions: his healthy core helps him cope with misfortunes. I wish one day we could discover the golden key to this group of IAPI children success, but for now, they remain an empirical fact defying boundaries and stereotypes.

Adoptive Families

Now let us consider the receiving side—adoptive families: what is the Point B for an adopted child? This analysis is based on the North American population, assuming that Western European adoptive parents possess similar characteristic. The majority (73%) of all international adoptees live with two married parents. About 4% live with lesbian or gay parents. A sizable minority of 23% lives in a single-parent household (Jones & Placek, 2017). With a very few exceptions, adoptive parents belong to the middle and upper middle class with average household earnings over 300% to 400% of the poverty level (National Center for Health Statistics, 2017). The overwhelming majority (95%) of international adoptees have parents with education above the high school level. Forty-three percent of adoptive parents of IAPI children are employed full time, the majority of the rest own businesses or are independent professionals. Nearly 96% of IAPI children live in middle-class neighborhoods, mostly in suburbia (Vandivere et al., 2009). All perspective adoptive parents went through a home-study process (state-regulated procedure for determining fitness for adoption, including health, criminal records, financial status, etc.). All adoptive parents had some training and education provided by their adoptive agency and other relevant agencies. Many belong to local and state volunteer groups of adoptive parents, and the majority participates in Internet-based discussion groups related to the donated country (Russia, China, Guatemala, etc.).

In about half of adoptive families, the adopted child is the first and only child with first-time parents. The rest, however, have biological children in the family, and those children are usually older than the adopted child. The mean age of adoptive mothers in the 2011 survey of kindergarteners in the US was 43 years, significantly higher than the 35-year-old average for mothers in families with both birth parents and higher than the 31-year-old average for mothers in single-parent and step families. The educational level of adoptive parents (53% being college graduates or having advanced degrees) was higher than the same in birth parents (42% graduated from a college). In terms of race and ethnicity, whites made up the majority of adoptive parents in the 2011 survey. Their proportion among the adoptive parents was significantly larger than the proportion of white children among the adopted children, implying that a substantial portion of the white parents were raising nonwhite children (Zill, 2017b).

In sum, individuals and couples who adopted internationally are mature in age, well-educated, financially well-to-do, and a strongly motivated group (Compton, 2016; Zill, 2017a). One more specific feature of adoptive parents: they are especially anxious and sensitive about their children's well-being and are forceful in obtaining needed treatment for them, seeking out expert care at the earliest sign of trouble (Hamilton, Cheng, & Powell, 2007).

It is informative to consider the adoptive family functioning through the lens of parental investment theory (Keller, Nesse, & Hofferth, 2001). This paradigm refers to the amount of time, energy, personal involvement, and material resources that parents put into caring for their children. From a human psychological prospective, the parental investment phenomenon includes economic, cultural, social, and interactional resources that parents provide for their children. Using data from the Early Childhood Longitudinal Study, Kindergarten-First Grade Waves (ECLS-K), Hamilton et al. (2007) studied data from 13,000 households and found that an adoptive family demonstrates advantages over all types of families, including the two-parent biological family. Thus, two-parent adaptive families invest in the most resources (financial, cultural, social, and interactional) at significantly higher levels than other types of families, thus enriching their children's lives to compensate for the lack of biological ties and the extra challenges of adoption.

There is one more factor that I call a "super-parenting drive," which is aptly explained by the so-called compensation theory—a strategy whereby one strives to compensate, consciously or unconsciously, for weaknesses, frustrations, desires, or feelings of inadequacy/incompetence in one area through gratification or drive toward excellence in another area. It suggests that a social context favoring biological parenthood creates disadvantages for adoptive parents, thus devaluing the social meaning of such a family as "not real" and "artificial" (Wegar, 2000). In order to overcome this bias, adoptive parents are trying to be "super parents," the "best parents possible," "ideal parents," "perfect parents," etc. They are doing this by increasing parental investment and in fact fully accomplish and even exceed expectations attributed by our culture to biological parents. Elevated sensitivity to their children's real or perceived needs forces adoptive parents to make a tremendous parental investment to rehabilitate and remediate their adopted children. Adoptive parents, being older than the majority of biological parents, start their parenthood with greater commitment and more preparation. According to the results of a national study, adoptive parents not only spend more money on their children, but they invest more time, such as reading to them, talking with their children about their problems, or eating meals together (Hamilton et al., 2007).

Now let us consider some less known and more controversial characteristics of adoptive parents, particularly their motivation to adopt. The motivation to adopt internationally has enormous significance for adoption as the process and the end result. It affects the capacity to withstand the difficulties of adoption, the perception of the outcome, and feelings and attitudes that accompany the whole process. According to one of the most comprehensive surveys (see A Chartbook Based on the 2007 National Survey of Adoptive Parents, US Department of Health and Human Services[12]), parents who adopted internationally listed the following as their major motivations for action:

- Desire to expand family,
- Wish to provide a permanent home and/or save a child,
- Infertility and need to have a child, or
- Wish to have a sibling for another child.

Like every attempt to quantify feelings, the above classifications are simplified. In real life, it's more often a combination of several reasons that urges people into action. To complement this four-point taxonomy the following is my classification of motivation to adopt, with some brief explanations. This information is based on nearly 30 years of interviewing actual adoptive parents who brought their children to my office for developmental, neuropsychological, and educational assessments.

Altruistic Egotism

"I want to be a parent. I want to love a child and be loved by a child." This is one of the most successful and positive motivations when adoptive parents aren't trying to prove anything to the world or to themselves; when, with no illusions of noble calling, they quietly pursue their own interests, a kind of Ayn Rand's objectivism applied to adoption. In the end everybody wins. This motivation rests upon the foundation of bare utilitarianism stripped of humanitarian high talk and altruistic bunk. The parents were using international adoption to achieve their own goals just to be parents. Egotism, in this case, must have had an underappreciated side if an openly self-centered stimulus could deliver such selfless results.

Answering the Divine Call

One of the most powerful motivators is faith, with multiple adoptions typically taking place in ultra-religious families that let this call be their driving force. The degree of success in such families varies. Sometimes it works out, sometimes it doesn't; when a tragic case with an international adoptee has been picked up by media (when kids were injured, mistreated, or even killed), to my surprise, a considerable percentage of such cases involved religious families. That rescue-at-any-cost mentality often lies at the root of dissatisfaction with the adoption experience and serves as the fundamental reason for an adoption fiasco. In general, this "save a child" motivation correlates with collapsed and/or extremely difficult adoptions, implying a rarely fulfilled appreciation from either the child or society. With no gratitude delivered, such adoption fails to live up to the ideal: the parents, "saviors and heroes" in their own eyes, set themselves up for trouble and tend to blame the children for that.

Loneliness

This is a complex and subjectively destructive feeling, determined by social, emotional, and spiritual factors. Not surprisingly, one of the most effective alternatives to medication in curing loneliness is a so-called pet-assisted therapy. However, adopting a child could be a means of coping with depressive loneliness. Looking to fill a void in their lives, some single parents treat their newly adopted children (in my experience, almost always a mother-daughter dyad) as an equal companion. Unfortunately, the hope that an adopted child will provide meaning to daily life and cure all ills is a classic pitfall. This is an unfair burden for any partner and especially inappropriate for a child who has no experience with parental bond or parental authority. Those who adopt to mend their loneliness often end up with an unbalanced parent-child relationship and attachment issues. When the mistake becomes apparent, these parents get disillusioned, feel sorry for themselves, and seek other solutions, forgetting that their soul-searching may have wrecked the life of another human being.

Stitching Together After Marital Ruptures

Having kids in order to save a family is the oldest trick in the book. Many cultures share the belief that a father would never abandon his offspring. A flavor of that belief found its way into adoption considerations.

Do as the Smiths Do

Adoption in our social solar system shares one physical quality with celestial bodies: gravity. People, who are more susceptible to such gravitational pull, may cross the boundary of what is known as the "point of no return" and underestimate their real desires and intentions. I know many families that initially did not plan an international adoption, as they already had their own two or three kids. However, out of curiosity, or following the pastor's plea during a Sunday sermon, a family signs up for a summer hosting program and spends three weeks with a 7-year-old girl or boy from an oversea orphanage. The parents fall in love with the hosted child and without much thinking or planning, the family members find themselves in the thick of adoption-related bustle. They socialize with others involved in adoption; they attend meetings organized by adoption agencies; they follow adoption blogs and share stories; they feel active, invigorated, and important. It's just a matter of time before they apply for an adoption of that child without really thinking through the whole situation.

Modus Vivendi

There is a group of people—not many, but more than one may suspect—who make adoption a major theme of their lives. They keep adopting from abroad, and the number of children in the family, often combined with the biological children, may exceed a dozen, or, as in two cases I know about, even reaching 18 and 19. To make sense of the big world, everyone creates a personal replica of the universe. These parents choose their social niche in the adoption community. Participating in reference groups, they share their problems and search for solutions. Adoption becomes their job and the meaning of life. Their virtual world is brimming with blogs. Their physical world rotates around get-togethers and conferences. At times, this lifestyle trespasses common sense (as elusive as its definition may be) and becomes an enclosed ecosystem. The larger the family, the higher the toll, demanding more time, more resources, invading the parents' every thought, and becoming their business, their faith, and their obsession: family, the whole family, and nothing but the family. It works for some and is not manageable or even acceptable for others.

Mental Ailment

After years of battling deep-seated personality issues, phobias, and neurotic fixations, with a hint from a therapist or following one's own insight, some people choose adoption to solve their mental health problems. As a rule, this choice is shielded by an outward motivation of saving a child or starting a family. Most attempts to discover these subtle, but powerful, mental disorders at the pre-adoption screening time are not successful, though there is a special section in the home study devoted the questions about mental health.

Whatever the motivation to adopt, the prospective adoptive parents have ideas and feelings for an "imaginary ideal child" who will be responsive to their care and love. What they have in reality is a child who has no idea what family life in a new country is all about, is in a survival mode of existence (and therefore is bound to test the limits for a very long time), and is resistant to care and distrustful of caregivers. Most adopted children rely on survival skills learned in orphanages, and those skills are incompatible with family life. My interactions for many years with prospective adoptive parents have led me to conclude that many, if not the majority of adoptive parents—whatever motivation they may have—possess unrealistic expectations and overly optimistic attitudes toward their planned endeavor. Many adoptive families and single parents planning an international adoption present a case of the "positivity bias," also known as "Pollyanna syndrome." (Boucher & Osgood, 1969). The name came from the 1913 novel *Pollyanna* by E. Porter, describing an orphan girl—how handy!—who was always cheerful and euphoric and perceived the world in the most positive way in spite of all misfortunes that happened to her. Unfortunately, "Pollyannaism" in the field of international adoption, created by adoption agencies (not always intentionally) and in part by media, facilitates unrealistic attitudes and romantic expectations related to international adoption. It often results in inadequate preparation, unrealistic attitudes, and improbable expectations associated with international adoption.

Adoption Outcomes

Adoptive parents apply extraordinary efforts, time, and patience simply to become one; with parents so dedicated and resourceful, why do adopted children seem to struggle so much, and why have so many adoptions failed? Why are there even difficulties and tragic outcomes from this arrangement along with obvious accomplishments and successes?

The wide range of motivations to adopt and other factors related to parental individual differences make adoptive families as diverse as the children they have adopted. A perfect match between an adopted child and an adoptive parent is illusive and random. Marriage is a good analogy: in developed countries, nearly every second marriage ends in divorce. What about the statistics of international adoption disruption and dissolution?

According to data from the federal Child Welfare Information Gateway (2012), up to 10% of international adoptions end up in what is called "disruption" or, using a popular euphemism, "re-homing." It means just one thing: in one out of ten adoptive families, the adoptive parents and the adopted child cannot live together anymore, and the parents initiate a "divorce" known as dissolution of adoption.

Sometimes the three terms—re-homing, disruption, and dissolution—are used interchangeably, even though each has its own specific meaning. Overall, according to Child Welfare Information Gateway (2012), the term "disruption" describes the situation in which the legal relationship between the adoptive parents and the adoptive child is severed, either voluntarily or involuntarily, after the adoption was legally finalized. This results in the child's placement with new adoptive parents (or temporary placement in the state custody). Typically, disruption happens due to the adoptive parents' inability to meet the child's needs within their family (Coakley & Berrick, 2008).

A few particularly bad endings in international adoption have made national news, including famous novelist Joyce Maynard's decision to give her two adopted Ethiopian girls to another family in 2012[13] and the Tennessee mother who put her adopted 7-year-old son back on a plane to his native Russia[14] in 2010. Even more tragic is the fact of legally confirmed deaths from the hands of adoptive parents of 19 adoptees from the former Soviet Union in the period from 1991 to 2016 (Miller, Chan, Reece, Tirella, & Pertman, 2007; Compton, 2016; Pound Pup Legacy organization[15]).

Clinical Case: Reggie—Disaster Beyond Repair

Brought from India to New Jersey at the age of 7 years, Reggie had no documented developmental history. Her adoptive parents were schoolteachers in their early 50s. Five years later, they retired and moved to Florida. Two more years later, when Reggie was 14 years old, the father passed away.

Academic and behavioral issues haunted Reggie from the very beginning. Initially homeschooled by her adoptive parents, she attended a parochial Catholic school and then public school, was classified as "learning disabled," and later as an "emotionally disturbed" student. Reggie spent most of her school time in special education.

I did a psychological evaluation of her three times: at the ages of 7, 12, and 16. A strong and physically active girl, she tested in the borderline range cognitively and delayed academically. But the most troublesome were her chronic post-traumatic reactions to her environment. Reggie had severe attachment issues with her parents and behaved with mixed maturity: at times like a 5-year-old throwing temper tantrums and at times like an experienced, grown-up woman.

With superhuman patience and dedication, her parents did everything possible from therapies, to different parental techniques, to school-related remediation, but it was all in vain. Reggie's mother had no doubts that her husband's cancer was facilitated by their unceasing stress with Reggie. The father's death coincided with the girl's sophomore year in high school, where her troubles turned into felonies. According to her mother, Reggie was desperate to fit in and yet not sophisticated enough to engage in age-appropriate interactions. She remained in survival mode, and for her, there was no past or future, only what she wanted at the current moment in time.

Reggie began stealing money and valuables from her family and classmates. She became sexually active before her 15th birthday. A few times, as a member of a local gang, Reggie was arrested and stayed in police custody overnight. When confronted, she grew violent and once hit her mother so badly that the woman had to be treated in a hospital. The letter that follows was not a plea for help but rather a cry of desperation.

I finally found strength to write you. It is all very bad. I got her, at last, to a psychiatrist, but she vehemently refused to take any medication. During all of her time in HS, before her expulsion, Reggie was stealing cell phones and other belongings of her classmates and got suspended several times from school. In November, I discovered that the entire year when she was taking the dog for a walk at 3 pm., she was really going to an apartment four blocks away and prostituting herself and exploiting herself via the stolen cell phones to a hardcore porn site (this is all in the police report). When I found out, she ran away from home. I took legal action against her and got a court order saying that she had to live at home, go to counseling, etc., or go to jail. She went to jail three times. She says she likes it there, as it is full of kids just like her, and she gets a free attorney "who talks to her." She was home on house arrest for four weeks in January, and it was torture. Reggie would swear at me nonstop, very foul mouthed. On one occasion, after five hours of swearing, I asked her if she wanted to play a board game, she said, "I want to split your f-king head open with an axe and smear your f-king brains on the floor." I am trying to save her from being thrown into jail, spending all my money on attorneys. She said to police that I have always been abusive to her and that I had driven her into the mountains and abandoned her barefoot in the snow. The most awful thing is that now she has a boyfriend who at 18 is a registered level 3 sex offender. He has three felonies and seven arrests, mostly as a juvenile but some as an adult. In July, she ran away from home with him and has been calling about every six to eight weeks and yelling and threatening to kill me, always from a restricted number. Finally, she said to me that she is six months pregnant. There is an active bench warrant here for her arrest, as she is in contempt of court, and she is running across the country with her boyfriend, moving from state to state. It is a very sad story; all I can do is pray, especially for the poor baby she is going to have. I fear for its safety. I have learned that, sad as it is, you can't help someone who doesn't want help. At times, I think she is a sociopath. I do believe she is capable of killing me.

This is a description of a child who is beyond our abilities to remediate and rehabilitate. Her formative years led to severe emotional trauma, canceling the positive aspect of development: the damage is irreversible and lasts a lifetime. In my clinical experience, dozens and dozens of cases prove that no efforts, no resources, not the best parenting and therapies can help save this category of children adopted from different countries, growing up mentally and emotionally unstable, unemployable, and homeless.

I sense an outrage against such a conclusion: defying odds is what makes us human; quitting is easy but persistence and perseverance create miracles. Alas, through no fault of their own, certain, a rather small, but still noticeable, set of IAPI children are sent down the one-way path. This assumption is hard to swallow, but children that belong to this category should never be adopted. They destroy the lives of those who try to help them and would be subjectively better off in their native environs.

There is a widespread conviction (see: Compton, 2016) that if a child is adopted before 5, as a toddler or, better yet, an infant, a team of caring parents and skilled professionals can surely interfere and prevent the downfall. The younger the child, the better his/her chances are to remold. Although this assumption seems reasonable, the age of adoption doesn't quite correlate with the results. Clinical data confirm that children adopted at as early as 3 or 4 months may still end up in the category described earlier. Despite all efforts, by their teenage years, they may demonstrate propensity for drugs, alcohol, and law violations.

There are many reasons that lead to adoption breakdown, and in most cases, this is an accumulation of interrelated and mutually influencing factors. Festinger (2002, 2014), gives a different disruption rate, varying from 9% to 15%, although among older children, he reports that the rate is even higher. (This is combined domestic and international adoption data.) Festinger pointed out that the primary factors associated with higher risk of disruption are as follows:

1. Children: their older age and more adversity prior to adoption cause more behavioral issues.
2. Parents: a lack of social support, particularly from relatives; unrealistic expectations; inadequate preparation; and a lack of prior adoptive or foster care experience.
3. Adoption-related social and mental health services characteristics: preparation for adoption is absent or very limited; scant information is given to the family about the child; after-adoption fragmented or disjointed services.

Significant difficulties accompany the process of international adoption, even when it does not result in formal dissolution. The rest of this book is devoted, in part, to the analysis of the "risk factors" in international adoption.

In conclusion, adoptive families, as well as orphanages, are heterogeneous entities. While we cannot consider institutions as a certified evil, we cannot accept the adoptive family as a guaranteed benevolent terminus for the IAPI children either. Both point A (institution) and point B (adoptive family) could be a source of adverse childhood experience; both could be a basis for resilience and growth. Both are human creations, and both are socially determined environments of a child's development.

International Adoption as a Unique "Natural Experiment"

Modern-day international adoption is a unique "natural experiment" in the study of child development. One of the central scientific issues of human development is how early life experiences affect physical growth, physiological maturity, and social adaptation of a human being. The opportunity to experimentally manipulate early human experiences is very limited for ethical reasons; thus, one approach is to observe a naturally occurring population of children who were reared in deficient environments. Analysis of specific delays and disorders in IAPI children allows us to find out how prenatal exposure to different teratogens (e.g., alcohol) prolongs severe social neglect and how other adverse childhood experiences may affect human growth and adaptation.

Adoptive families provide a critical case for investigating the mechanisms of parenting outside the context of biological kinship. Actually, it may tell us about the origin of parental capacity itself: is it a biological instinct or psychological desire, or a mix of both and how does one mediate the other?

From the cultural perspective of psychology, international adoption allows more closely examined evidence regarding how children are affected when reared in a family and culture that differs from that of their biological ancestors. Do we observe cultural confusion that negatively affects development and emotional well-being, or are children able to establish healthy identities and a strong sense of belongingness to social groups in their country of rearing? Can particular parenting strategies, community characteristics, or adoption practices support the development of a strong sense of identity in internationally adopted children and adults?

Research in the field of international adoption gives a new impulse to attachment theory and therapeutic practices, with its focus on early human connectedness and the adverse consequences of the lack of it for future development.

Research on first-language attrition in international adoptees sheds light on the nature of bilingualism, on the origin of certain language pathologies (e.g., language attrition in aphasia) and on causal mechanisms underlying differences in the language acquisition process.

In my professional opinion, the most significant contribution of international adoption as a natural experiment is seen in the field of complex childhood trauma. Internationally adopted orphans comprise the extreme group of individuals whose development has been mediated by complex childhood trauma. Scientific research of their development under stress, whether prenatal, postnatal, during the adoption transition, or in post-adoption life can provide us with discoveries that could be extrapolated to all children who experience severe adversity in their life. We cannot ignore the opportunities presented by studying adopted children and adoptive families. International adoption in its role of "natural experiment" provides us with a wealth of data that needs to be properly understood.

BGCenter Statistics of Clinical Data

In my database, there are 766 clinical cases: the full combined developmental, neuropsychological, and educational assessments (in the English language), and the screenings upon arrival, done in the child's native language. There are two types of assessments:

- A screening upon arrival (usually within 10 days to 30 days after landing in the US or Canada). Screening is done in the native language (Russian and Ukrainian by this writer, while screening in Chinese and Spanish was performed by certified school psychologists, native speakers of the targeted languages, under direct supervision and in collaboration with this author). Several screenings were completed with participation of a translator from such languages as Amharic (Ethiopia), Armenian, Bulgarian, Latvian, Polish, and Hungarian. A sample of testing procedures used during screening is presented in **Addendum 1**.
- A combined developmental, neuropsychological, and educational assessment in the English language is performed after at least two years of the child's life in the US or Canada. A sample of testing procedures used during such assessment is presented in **Addendum 2**.

Age and gender: All cases in the database represent children from ages 4 to 18 years. The bulk of all the examinees (over 75%) is in the age group from 6 to 13. Gender is generally congruent with the overall adoption statistics: our database contains 56% female cases and 44% male cases.

The following countries were represented in our database: Russian Federation and the former Soviet republics (Ukraine, Kazakhstan, Kirgizstan, Moldova, Latvia, Estonia, Armenia): 64% of all cases; China: 16%; Latin America (Guatemala, Colombia, Peru, Ecuador): 8%; Eastern Europe Romania, Poland, Bulgaria, and Hungary: 8%; India: 1%; Ethiopia: 1%; Philippines: 1%; and other countries: 1% (e.g., Albania and Vietnam).

One big advantage of my clinical work is that I have access to the legal (court documents), medical, and developmental (medical records) and even educational (school grades and school files) documentation for most of the examined children, and, rarely, even psychological and educational assessment summaries from the native countries. This documentation has its own limitations and biases, of course, but still, that information was not available to most of the researchers in the field of international adoption. It creates a valuable context for the interpretation of clinical data. Numerous interviews with adoptive parents and participation in online discussions and conferences provide still another source of information.

In this book, the reader meets with several descriptions of the real-life cases, illustrating some thoughts and findings in my clinical practice. In order to protect the identity of my patients, in these stories, I changed the names and countries of origin of the children, and, sometimes, certain details that may identify the individual. There is only one exception: the letters written by Reggie's mother and Diana's mother, which are original and only slightly shortened. I have written permission from both clients to publish these messages.

Notes

1. https://travel.state.gov/content/travel/en/Intercountry-Adoption/adopt_ref/ adoption-statistics.html and https://travel.state.gov/content/travel/en/ Intercountry-Adoption.html
2. https://travel.state.gov/content/travel/en/Intercountry-Adoption/adopt_ref/ adoption-statistics.html
3. www.cdc.gov/nchs/slaits/nsap.htm
4. www.schusterinstituteinvestigations.org/
5. www.hcch.net/en/instruments/conventions/full-text/?cid=69
6. https://travel.state.gov/content/dam/aa/pdfs/2015NarrativeAnnualReporton IntercountryAdoptions.pdf
7. www.uscis.gov/tools/glossary/orphan
8. https://legal-dictionary.thefreedictionary.com/adoption
9. www.adoptioninstitute.org/old/publications/2010_10_20_KeepingThe Promise.pdf
10. Retrieved October 7, 2017, from https://twitter.com/jk_rowling/status/ 773967096745263104
11. www.youtube.com/watch?v=VCeWr8OFuEs
12. http://aspe.hhs.gov/hsp/09/nsap/chartbook/chartbook.cfm?id=1
13. http://hereandnow.legacy.wbur.org/2013/10/09/maynard-adopted-children
14. www.cnn.com/2012/07/13/us/adopted-child-returned/
15. http://poundpuplegacy.org/about

References

Adoption Disruption and Dissolution. (2012). *Child welfare information gateway.* Retrieved from https://www.childwelfare.gov/pubs/s_disrup.cfm

Adoption USA: A Chartbook Based on the 2007 National Survey of Adoptive Parents. (2007). *US department of health and human services.* Retrieved from http://aspe.hhs.gov/hsp/09/nsap/chartbook/chartbook.cfm?id=1

Bakermans-Kranenburg, M., Van Jzendoorn, M., & Juffer, E. (2008). Earlier is better: A meta-analysis of 70 years of interventions improving cognitive development in institutionalized children. *Monographs of the Society for Research of Child Development, 73*, 279–293.

Beckett, C., Castle, J., Rutter, M., & Sonuga-Barke, E. (2010). Institutional deprivation, specific cognitive functions, and scholastic achievement: English and Romanian Adoptee (ERA) study findings. *Monographs of the Society for Research in Child Development, 75*, 125–142.

Boucher, J., & Osgood, C. (1969). The Pollyanna hypothesis. *Journal of Verbal and Learning Behavior, 8*(1), 1–8.

Bureau of Consular Affairs, U.S. Department of State Statistics. (2016). Retrieved from https://travel.state.gov/content/dam/NEWadoptionassets/pdfs/AnnualRep ortonIntercountryAdoptions6.8.17.pdf

Child Adoption: Trends and Policies. (2009). *Report of UN department of economic and social affairs* (p. XV). Retrieved from www.un.org/esa/population/publications/adoption2010/child_adoption.pdf

Clark, P., Thigpen, S., & Moeller-Yates, A. (2006). Integrating the older/special needs adoptive child into the family. *Journal of Marital and Family Therapy, 32*(2), 181–194.

Coakley, J. F., & Berrick, J. D. (2008). Research review: In a rush to permanency: Preventing adoption disruption. *Child and Family Social Work, 13*, 101–112.

Compton, R. (2016). *Adoption beyond borders: How international adoption benefits children.* New York: Oxford University Press.

Dubrovina, I. (1991). *Psychological development of children in orphanages* (Psichologicheskoe razvitie vospitanikov v detskom dome). Moscow: Prosveschenie Press. (In the Russian language).

Ela, E. J. (2011). *Adoption motivations among U.S. parents: National Center for Family and Marriage Research (NCFMR) tabulations based on 2007 national survey of adoptive parents.* Publication by Bowling Green State University Scholar Works. Retrieved from http://scholarworks.bgsu.edu/cgi/viewcontent.cgi?article=1000&context=ncfmr_family_profiles

Evan Donaldson Adoption Institute. (2010). Keeping the promise: The critical need for post-adoption services to enable children and families to succeed. *Policy & Practice Perspective.* Retrieved from www.adoptioninstitute.org/old/publications/2010_10_20_KeepingThePromise.pdf

Festinger, T. (2002). After adoption: Dissolution or permanence? *Child Welfare, 81*(3), 515–533.

Festinger, T. (2014). Adoption disruption: Rates, correlates, and service needs. In G. P. Mallon & P. M. Hess (Eds.), *Child welfare for the 21st century: A handbook of practices, policies, and programs* (2nd ed.). New York: Columbia University Press.

Ford, T., Vostanis, P., Meltzer, H., & Goodman, R. (2007). Psychiatric disorder among British children looked after by local authorities: Comparison with children living in private households. *British Journal of Psychiatry, 190*, 319–325.

Gindis, B. (2005). Cognitive, language, and educational issues of children adopted from overseas orphanages. *Journal of Cognitive Education and Psychology, 4*(3), 290–315.

Goodwin, D. K. (1994). *No ordinary time.* New York: Simon & Shuster.

Graff, E. (2009, November/December). The lie we love. *Foreign Policy Magazine*. Retrieved from http://foreignpolicy.com/2009/10/06/the-lie-we-love/

Graff, E. (2010a). Anatomy of adoption crisis. *Foreign Policy Magazine*. Retrieved from http://foreignpolicy.com/2010/09/12/anatomy-of-an-adoption-crisis/

Graff, E. (2010b). The baby business. *Democracy Journal*. Retrieved from https://democracyjournal.org/magazine/17/the-baby-business/

Gunnar, M. (2001). Effects of early deprivation. In C. Nelson & M. Luciana (Eds.), *Handbook of developmental cognitive neuroscience* (pp. 617–629). Cambridge, MA: The MIT Press.

Hamilton, L., Cheng, S., & Powell, B. (2007). Adoptive parents, adaptive parents: Evaluating the importance of biological ties for parental investment. *American Sociological Review*, 72(1), 95–116.

Hjern, A., Lindblad, F., & Vinnerljung, B. (2002). Suicide, psychiatric illness, and social maladjustment in intercountry adoptees in Sweden: A cohort study. *Lancet*, 360(9331), 443–448.

Ji, J., Brooks, D., Barth, R., & Kim, H. (2010). Beyond pre-adoptive risk: The impact of adoptive family environment on adopted youth's psychosocial adjustment. *American Journal of Orthopsychiatry*, 80(3), 432–442.

Johnson, D. (2000). Medical and developmental sequelae of early childhood institutionalization in Eastern European adoptees. In C. Nelson (Ed.), *The effects of early adversity on neurobehavioral development: Minnesota symposium on child psychology* (Vol. 31, pp. 113–162). Mahwah, NJ: Lawrence Erlbaum Associates.

Johnston, R. (2017). Historical international adoption statistics. *United States and World*. Retrieved April 2017, from www.johnstonsarchive.net/policy/adoptionstatsintl.html

Jones, J., & Placek, P. (2017). *Adoption by the numbers*. A Comprehensive Report of US Adoption Statistics, Publication of National Council for Adoption (NCFA). Retrieved from: https://indd.adobe.com/view/4ae7a823-4140-4f27-961a-cd9f16a5f362

Juffer, F., Palacios, J., LeMare, L., Sonuga-Barke, E., Tieman, W., & Bakermans-Kranenburg, M. (2012). Development of adopted children with histories of early adversity. In R. McCall, M. Van lJzendoorn, F. Juffer, V. Groza, & C. Groark (Eds.), *Children without permanent parental care: Research, practice, and policy*. Monographs of the Society for Research of Child Development. Hoboken, NJ, USA: Wiley-Blackwell Publishing.

Keiger, D. (1996, April). The rise and demise of the American Orphanage. *John Hopkins Magazine*. Retrieved May 2018, from http://pages.jh.edu/jhumag/496web/orphange.html

Keller, M. C., Nesse, R. M., & Hofferth, S. (2001). The Trivers-Willard hypothesis of parental investment: No effect in contemporary United States. *Evolution and Human Behavior*, 22, 343–360.

MacLean, K. (2003). The impact of institutionalization on child development. *Development and Psychopathology*, 15, 853–884.

McCall, J. (1998). Research on the psychological effects of orphanage care: A critical review. In R. McKenzie (Ed.), *Rethinking orphanages for the 21st century*. Thousand Oaks, CA: Sage Publications.

Miller, L. (2005). *The handbook of international adoption medicine: A guide for physicians, parents, and providers*. Oxford, UK: Oxford University Press.

Miller, L., Chan, W., Reece, R., Tirella, L., & Pertman, A. (2007). Child abuse fatalities among internationally adopted children. *Child Maltreatment, 12*(4), 378–380.

Morison, S. J., & Ellwood, A. L. (2000). Resiliency in the aftermath of deprivation: A second look at the development of Romanian orphanage children. *Merrill-Palmer Quarterly, 46*(4), 717–737.

National Center for Health Statistics. (2017). Adoption and nonbiological parenting trend table. Key Statistics from the NSFG. Retrieved from www.cdc.gov/nchs/nsfg/key_statistics/a.htm

Pertman, A. (2011). *Adoption nation* (2nd ed.). Boston, MA: Harvard Common Press.

Pinderhughes, E., Matthews, J., Deoudes, G., & Pertman, A. (2013). *A changing world: Shaping best practices through understanding of the new realities of intercountry adoption.* Publication of the Donaldson Adoption Institute. Retrieved from https://adoptioninstitute.org/old/publications/2013_10_AChangingWorld.pdf

Rutter, M. (1999). Resilience concepts and findings: Implications for family therapy. *Journal of Family Therapy, 21*, 119–144.

Rutter, M., Kreppner, J. M., & O'Connor, T. G. (2001). Specificity and heterogeneity in children's responses to profound institutional privation. *The British Journal of Psychiatry, 179*, 97–103.

Rutter, M., Sonuga-Barke, E. J. S., Beckett, C., Castle, J., Kreppner, J., Kumsta, R., & Bell, C. A. (2010). Deprivation-specific psychological patterns: Effects of institutional deprivation. *Monographs of the Society for Research in Child Development,* Serial No. 295, *75*(1).

Selman, P. (2009). The rise and fall of intercountry adoption in the 21st century. *International Social Work, 52*(5), 575–594.

Selman, P. (2012). *Global trends in intercountry adoption: 2001–2010* (Adoption Advocate, #44). Publication of National Council for Adoption.

Shipitsyna, L. (2008). *Psychology of orphans.* Bloomington, IN: iUniverse Publisher.

The St. Petersburg-USA Orphanage Research Team. (2009). The effects of early social-emotional and relationship experience on the development of young orphanage children. *Monographs of the Society for Research in Child Development, 73*(3), vii–295. Publisher: John Wiley & Sons.

Turner-Strong, P. (2001). To forget their tongue, their name, and their whole relation. In S. Franklin & S. McKinnon (Eds.), *Relative values: Reconfiguring kinship studies* (pp. 468–493). Durham, NC: Duke University Press.

US Department of State. (n.d.). https://travel.state.gov/content/travel/en/Intercountry-Adoption/adopt_ref/adoption-statistics.html

US Department of State. (2014). *Annual report on intercountry adoption.* Retrieved from https://travel.state.gov/content/dam/aa/pdfs/fy2013_annual_report.pdf

US State Department. (2017). *Immigrant visas issued to orphans coming to the US.* Retrieved from www.passportsusa.com/family/adoption/stats/stats_451.html

Valeeva, R., & Kalimulin, M. (2015). Social orphanhood in Russia: Historical background, present and perspective. *Procedia: Social and Behavioral Sciences, 191*(2), 2122–2126.

Van den Dries, L., Juffer, F., Van IJzendoorn, M., & Bakermans-Kranenburg, M. (2009). Fostering security? A meta-analysis of attachment in adopted children. *Children and Youth Services Review, 31*, 410–421.

Vandivere, S., Malm, K., & Radel, L. (2009). *Adoption USA: A chartbook based on the 2007 National Survey of adoptive parents.* US Department of Health and Human Services.

Van IJzendoorn, M. H., Bakermans-Kranenburg, M. J., & Juffer, F. (2007). Plasticity of growth in height, weight and head circumference: Meta-analytic evidence for massive catch-up after international adoption. *Journal of Developmental and Behavioral Pediatrics, 28*(4), 334–343.

Van IJzendoorn, M. H., & Juffer, F. (2005a). Adoption is a successful natural intervention enhancing adopted children's IQ and school performance. *Current Directions in Psychological Science, 14*(6), 319–329.

Van IJzendoorn, M. H., & Juffer, F. (2005b). Behavior problems and mental health referrals of international adoptees: A meta-analysis. *Journal of the American Medical Association, 293*, 2501–2515.

Van IJzendoorn, M. H., & Juffer, F. (2006). The Emanuel Miller memorial lecture: Adoption as intervention: Meta-analytic evidence for massive catch-up and plasticity in physical, socio-emotional, and cognitive development. *Journal of Child Psychology and Psychiatry, 47*(12), 1228–1245.

Van IJzendoorn, M. H., Palacios, J., Sonuga-Barke, E., Gunnar, M., Vorria, P., McCall, R., . . . Juffer, F. (2011). Children in institutional care: Delayed development and resilience. *Monographs of the Society for Research in Child Development, 76*(4), 8–30.

Wegar, K. (2000). Adoption, family ideology, and social stigma: Bias in community attitudes, adoption research, and practice. *Family Relations, 49*, 363–370.

Whitten, K. L., & Weaver, S. R. (2010). Adoptive family relationships and healthy adolescent development: A risk and resilience analysis. *Adoption Quarterly, 13*(3/4), 209–226.

Wright, L., & Flynn, C. (2006). Adolescent adoption: Success despite challenges. *Children & Youth Services Review, 28*(5), 489–490.

Zill, N. (2017a). The changing face of adoption in the United States. *Publication of Institute for Family Studies.* Retrieved from https://ifstudies.org/blog/the-changing-face-of-adoption-in-the-united-states

Zill, N. (2017b). Analysis of data from the Early Childhood Longitudinal Study of the Kindergarten Class of 2010–2011. *National Center for Education Statistics, U.S. Department of Education.* Retrieved from https://ifstudies.org/blog/the-changing-face-of-adoption-in-the-united-states

2 Developmental Trauma Disorder and Internationally Adopted Post-Institutionalized Children

Introduction

In the last 30 years, there has been an upsurge of publications on the psychopathology in children and adolescents related to their early childhood traumatic experiences. There is no need to reiterate the findings and theoretical postulations presented in the works of B. van der Kolk, P. Ogden, A. Shore, B. Perry, E. Tronick, their associates, and many other experts in the field. In this book, the concept of a complex relational childhood trauma is considered in the context of one special group of children: former residents of overseas orphanages who were adopted by North American families. The study of this contingent of children has significant practical application and important scientific value: internationally adopted children are the exemplum of development mediated by complex childhood trauma that reveals itself in how these children feel, think, learn at school, regulate their behavior, and socialize with their peers and adults. Understanding the critical interactions of neurodevelopmental and psychosocial processes in IAPI children is the current scientific frontier for researchers seeking to intervene in the effects of prolonged child maltreatment.

The Concept of Developmental Trauma Disorder

Although the very notion of trauma during early years of development and its consequences in human life is not a new theme in psychology and psychiatry, it is only at the beginning of the new millennium that the most comprehensive, systematic, multidisciplinary, and focused paradigm of adverse early childhood experiences was introduced by a group of psychologists and psychiatrists under the leadership of B. van der Kolk (2003, 2005, 2015). Multiple and long-term traumatic conditions and events, often against the background of neurological weaknesses and impairments, result in distorted neurodevelopment, designated as developmental trauma disorder (DTD). The concept of DTD was presented to the research and clinical community as a complex somatic and neuropsychological phenomenon, which is chronic, relational (caused by humans), and significant enough to affect the development of a child (D'Andrea, Ford, Stolbach, Spinazzola, & van der Kolk, 2012).

Researchers and practitioners in the field of mental health came to understand that continuous repetitive traumatic experiences during childhood produce a wide range of distortions in development. Still, the concept of complex childhood trauma is not uniform and homogeneous, which is reflected in terminology: current terms being used include "adverse childhood experience," "prolonged traumatic stress," "repetitive traumatization," "recurring distress," "complex childhood trauma," "relational childhood trauma," "early trauma," "complex PTSD," etc. (Tedeschi & Calhoun, 2004; Cook, et al., 2005; McCrory, De Brito, & Viding, 2010; Benjet, Borges, Mendez, Fleiz, & Medina-Mora, 2011; D'Andrea et al., 2012; Weinhold & Weinhold, 2015). All these terms describe both the child's exposure to multiple traumatic events and the wide-ranging, long-term impact of this exposure. What is common for all these notions, although in different degrees and emphasis, is that

- it is a prolonged, repetitive, often still ongoing occurrence(s);
- it has distinct interpersonal nature: a lack of security and stability in relationship with a caregiver(s) results in subjectively significant psychological and physiological stress;
- there are long-lasting negative consequences, both physiological and psychological, affecting the child, the family, and society; and
- at different stages of development, traumatic experience is processed differently and produces different outcomes: a developmental aspect is crucial in understanding and addressing DTD.

The following definition of DTD, which I have assembled from different sources, may serve as common ground in understanding what mediates the development of IAPI children: *Early childhood trauma is a condition caused by repetitive, pervasive, subjectively highly stressful events, mostly within the interpersonal context of the child' life that have an adverse, wide-ranging, and long-term physiological and psychological impact on the development and maturation of high psychological functions, thus compromising neurodevelopmental integration of sensory, emotional, and cognitive systems into cohesive whole of a mature socially adjusted individual.*

Please note that developmental trauma disorder (DTD) is not presented in current Diagnostic and Statistical Manual of Mental Disorders, 5th edition, 2013 (DSM 5) as the psychiatric diagnosis.

DTD is rooted and formed mostly before the child has the verbal and reasoning ability to process and store the traumatic experience in memory, thus the central nervous system (CNS) and physical body accumulate the traumatic reminiscences as somatic distress and afflictions. *The Body*

Keeps the Score, the title of van der Kolk's book (2015), explains how social stress turns into somatic (physiological) matter.

Human beings in the early stages of their development are extremely vulnerable to adversities that may have lifelong negative consequences for emotional regulation, biological arousal systems, attention/concentration, social connectedness, and other psychophysiological functions (Shonkoff & Garner, 2012). If the trauma persists in duration, intensity, or frequency, it can lead to permanent physiological and psychological changes: the biochemistry of the whole organism is affected in a significant and, in some cases, permanent way. The neurological research shows to what extent trauma affects a child on a biological and hormonal level, as well as psychologically and behaviorally; it is truly a complex mixture of biological, psychological, and social phenomena (Rothschild, 2000; Ogden, Minton, & Pain, 2006). If not addressed, DTD can distort the developmental trajectory for the remainder of the individual's life span, being linked to a wide range of problems, including addiction, chronic physical conditions, depression and anxiety, self-harming behaviors, and other psychiatric disorders. Beyond the consequences for the child and family, these problems carry high costs for society (Putnam, 2006).

An infant who has been abandoned by birth parents or lived in an extremely dysfunctional family, traumatized by life in an orphanage, and then adopted by strangers into a different sociocultural environment is at exceptional risk for DTD. In my opinion, based on 30 years of clinical experience and study of research literature, each and every IAPI child does have DTD to some extent—ranging in degree from overwhelming and incurable to mild and recoverable, but no survivor of this abnormal background escapes it without consequences.

Primary Physiological Trauma as a Contributing Factor of DTD

The physiological components of DTD in IAPI children develop *in utero* and go on during the pre-adoptive years and beyond. There is significant research literature on this matter, with the pinnacle of quality reached in a comprehensive volume written single-handedly by a veteran of adoption medicine, Dr. Laura Miller (2005), titled *The Handbook of International Adoption Medicine*. Its main idea is that practically all international adoptees, although to a different degree, suffer from primary (biological) trauma caused by encephalopathies of different etiologies related to prenatal conditions, birth circumstances, and adverse postnatal physical environments. In many IAPI children, the primary trauma is so substantial (e.g., in the case of fetal alcohol syndrome disorder—FASD) that their entire further development is affected by it.

My review of the medical documentation of 766 international adoptees from Eastern Europe, Latin America, China, and Africa revealed that the vast majority of birth mothers never had prenatal care. The same finding was reported in a number of medical publications (Miller, 2005; Mather, Bridgewater, Way, & Haworth, 2017). The majority of births took place in local hospitals, but a sizable minority of children were born either at home or in some shelters provided by churches or volunteer organizations. According to legal adoption documentation from Eastern Europe and countries of the former Soviet Union, the majority of IAPI children's birth mothers had several of the following conditions:

- Had chronic health problems
- Suffered from ongoing venereal diseases (most often syphilis) or were HIV-positive
- Abused alcohol (thus, according to the BGCenter statistics, over 10% among Russian biological mothers were officially designated as "certified alcoholic" while close to 75% of the remaining mothers were described as "abusing alcohol")
- Smoked during pregnancy
- Used narcotics
- Lived in an extreme impoverished environment
- Were exposed for a long time to various toxins (lead and other heavy metals, polluted air and water, etc.)
- Suffered from a long list of infections, including those practically eliminated in the modern Western countries diseases as tuberculosis
- Were malnourished or suffered from chronic hunger

The biological mothers of IAPI children are an extreme example of what is known as "social gradient in health" phenomenon (see "Social Determinants of Health," World Health Organization, 2008[1]). The social determinants of health are the circumstances in which people are born, grow up, and live. There is a social gradient in health that runs from the top to the bottom of the socioeconomic spectrum: research shows that, in general, the lower the individual's socioeconomic position, the worse their health is. Lower social class is associated with an increased risk of adverse health outcomes (Marmot & Wilkinson, 1999).

Medical conditions of international adoptees vary widely from country to country and even from region to region in the same country. Based on a significant volume of research and practice-oriented literature in the specialized field of international adoption medicine (Miller, 2005), the following trauma-contributing biological conditions could be identified as statistically prevalent in IAPI children as a group:

- Prenatal exposure to toxins (alcohol, lead, infections, etc.)
- Prematurity: the number of IAPI children who were born premature exceeds the average in the general population by four times (Miller, 2005). The negative consequences of extreme prematurity for

physical, academic, and social functioning are well known (Barclay, 2005)

- Birth-related injuries with known neurological aftereffects (e.g., hypoxia)
- Extremely low birth weight even in full-term babies: low birth weight highly correlates with learning and social difficulties during school years (Rodrigues, Mello, & Fonceca, 2006)
- Failure-to-thrive (FTT) condition: it is often, if not typical, for IAPI children adopted before their second birthday to have a condition known as failure-to-thrive (ICD-10 Code R62.51)—an obstruction to achieve typical physical standards during the first three years of life. An FTT diagnosis is usually based on the dynamic of the anthropometric measurements of weight, height, head, and chest circumferences taken every three to six months from birth to the age of 3 years. Feeding problems and social neglect are most often the causes of the FTT in IAPI children (Miller, 2005). As stated by the World Health Organization (Onis & Yip, 1996, p. 74), "*Growth assessment is the single measurement that best defines the health and nutritional status of children, just as it provides an indirect measurement of the quality of life of entire populations*"
- Long-term consequences of different perinatal encephalopathies with well-known (lead, alcohol, narcotics, infections, etc.) and unknown teratogens
- "Intrauterine growth retardation" (IUGR), a condition in which an unborn baby is smaller than it should be because it is not growing at a normal rate inside the womb. IUGR can be symmetrical (all parameters of growth are delayed) or asymmetrical (for example, normal length with the weight deficit). Symmetrical IUGR is caused by extreme fetal malnutrition and/or any condition causing restriction in growth potential, such as congenital infections, genetic disorders, and environmental toxins (including nicotine and alcohol). IUGR is not an equivalent of prematurity, both premature and full-term infants can have IUGR

In addition to the aforementioned, Miller (2005) points out a long list of other less frequent medical conditions among international adoptees.

A separate issue is the quality of medical documentation from the donating countries. Medical documentation of newly arrived adoptees varied tremendously from country to country in terms of the amount of information and its reliability. According to Miller's review (2005), the most accurate and informative were medical documentations from South Korea and the Russian Federation, and the least useful and revealing were from Ethiopia and India, with other countries being in the wide range of utility of their medical documentation. Most medical reports consisted of a basic physical examination and a list of inoculations, accompanied, at times, with a brief screening for important medical conditions. Virtually, no assessment of development was provided (Mather et al., 2017).

Beyond the amount of information and its accuracy in the foreign medical records, there were two factors that reduced their usefulness. First, all medical records from the donating countries are subject to translation, which produces substantial risk for errors and distortions. Second, there are some medical diagnoses, clinical procedures, and means of treatment that are not familiar to many American and Canadian pediatricians.

Particular debates are caused by a diagnosis of "perinatal encephalopathy" found in many medical records of children adopted from the states of the former Soviet Union and Eastern Europe[2]. Perinatal encephalopathy (literally "birth-related impairment") is a broad "catchall" term indicating that the child is medically "at risk." This diagnosis relates to risk factors present in the history of the mother (e.g., alcohol or substance abuse) and/or the child (e.g., low birth weight, prematurity, etc.) that may result in a poor neurological outcome[3]. In ICD-10-CM, one can readily find codes for specific perinatal encephalopathies (e.g., P91.63—severe hypoxic ischemic encephalopathy or P91.819—neonatal encephalopathy, unspecified), but still for many pediatricians in North America, it is a "foreign" diagnosis.

The fact is that the diagnosis of perinatal encephalopathy does not have steady, unwavering predictive validity for further development, and some children can be completely rehabilitated or compensated for. In other cases, however, it may result in a neurological condition known as *static encephalopathy, unspecified (ICD-10 Diagnosis Code G93.40)*. This condition, which in most cases is caused by an unknown agent, means a generalized weakness (dysregulation) of the CNS that encompasses a range of delays of varying magnitudes in different domains, particularly in the social/behavioral and cognitive areas.

In spite of many deficiencies and inaccuracies, just ignoring or dismissing medical diagnoses from donated country as "inaccurate," "exaggerated," or "weird" is the wrong way to go. These medical records still deserve attention and may contain information crucial to providing proper care for adopted children.

Secondary Trauma in IAPI Children

The secondary trauma in IAPI children is social in nature. It is produced by adverse social circumstances: dysfunctional and abusive family, total abandonment, institutionalization, international adoption, and post-adoption stress. At different stages of development—infant/toddler, preschooler, school-age "older" adoptee, adoption of adolescents—the secondary trauma reveals itself in various forms and degrees.

Let us look at possible and objectively traumatic events that are typical for the IAPI children's pre-adoption experience. Not all children live through these trauma-producing events or experience them in the same intensity; however, this list is not all inclusive either.

- Total abandonment (being "refused" at birth or fully relinquished within the first three to six months of life)
- Repeated desertion (being frequently left alone for many hours/days) during early childhood
- Sudden death or permanent severe physical/mental impairment of a primer caregiver
- Repeated change/separation from caregivers due to multiple placements
- Failed adoption or foster care attempt(s)
- Extreme physical discomfort: hunger, cold, dehydration, etc.
- Total neglect of basic physical and emotional needs
- Physical abuse: beating and torturing by primary caregiver(s) or other individuals
- Direct or indirect sexual abuse: rape or exposure to inappropriate sexual scenes
- Witnessing violence, physical assault, murder, fight, beating, and drinking/sexual orgies
- Placement in institution (an orphanage or hospital)
- Chronic illness, physical disability, dysmorphic features, specific handicapping condition(s)
- Repeated transfer between different institutions: orphanages, "sanatoriums," hospitals, etc.
- All kind of abuse by peers and older children in an orphanage (bullying, rape, teasing, etc.)
- Adoption to a foreign country: sudden loss of language, culture, physical environment

Contrary to common opinion, the change from an objectively adverse pre-adoption social situation of development to an objectively favorable post-adoption life does not cut the chain of traumatic impacts in IAPI children. Adjustment to a new physical, cultural, social, and linguistic environment is a traumatic encounter by itself: the old traumatic experience forms the background, but the new trauma of not fitting in, not being connected with, and not being accepted by the new social milieu creates a new and more subjectively genuine trauma. The long-lasting consequences of early traumatization continue to affect development but are now mediated by the mounting challenges of adjustment to and competition in a new social/cultural environment.

Now when an IAPI child is a part of American family, he or she is subjected to the same chances of hardship and misfortune as their non-adopted peers. Based on the 2016 Survey of Children's Health[4], two researchers, V. Sacks and D. Murphey, published an investigation, "The Prevalence of Adverse Childhood Experiences, Nationally, by

State, and by Race or Ethnicity," to determine which children 17 years and under are more likely to experience trauma and where these children live[5]. The authors listed eight different categories of adversity that objectively may qualify as potentially traumatic experience in a child:

- Parental divorce or separation
- Parental death
- Parental incarceration
- Violence among adults in the home
- Victim or witness to neighborhood violence
- Living with a mentally ill adult
- Living with someone who has a substance abuse problem
- Experiencing economic hardship often, such as difficulty affording food and housing

The authors found that, one in every ten children nationally has experienced three or more of these adverse childhood experiences (ACEs). In other words, after adoption, one out of ten IAPI child has a chance to live through the adverse childhood experiences listed above. I believe that among those ACEs listed by V. Sacks and D. Murphey, adoptive parental divorce and parental death are the two prevailing family-related, trauma-produced adversities in IAPI child after adoption.

There are certain factors that mediate the impacts of those events and conditions on an IAPI child, such as the age of the child, the intensity and duration of adverse experience, and the resilience forces (a counter-balance to traumatic impact). Thus, personality traits can support resilience or create vulnerabilities that limit adaptation and foster chronic impairment. Social support can have a dramatic effect on children's adaptation to traumatic stress. The overall state of a child's CNS is a factor affecting the onset, duration, or severity of the trauma effect. Please see more detailed discussion in the section called "Resilience to the Consequences of DTD in IAPI Children."

The Synergetic Effect of Multiple Sources of DTD in Internationally Adopted Children

There are many factors in a life story of an IAPI child that cause, sustain, and contribute to the formation of DTD. For theoretical speculation or even for a practical purpose of making a diagnosis and creating recommendations for treatment, we can separate these factors as "mostly physiological" and "mostly psychological." In reality, however, we are dealing with a synergetic effect of those deeply intertwined and closely interconnected components. Indeed, physiological encephalopathies could be aggravated by the social conditions of their existence to the extent of permanent psychiatric and/or somatic disorders. On the other hand, social circumstances and conditions could be exacerbated by the neurological weaknesses and impairments. The opposite is also true: physiological maladies could be compensated and remediated by the psychological means of rehabilitation, and adverse social circumstances may be less devastating in the case of healthy and resilient neurology.

Contemporary research suggests that social interactions or the lack thereof may affect neuroendocrine development, which can alter observed behaviors. Behavior in turn produces social feedback, which stimulates a neuroendocrine response and, being strong enough, may cause modifications in neural structures: relations become biological structure (Perry, Pollard, Blakely, Baker, & Vigilante, 1995; Mehta, Golembo, & Nosarti, 2009). In other words, this action is bidirectional: the genes and the epigenetic modifications in their transcription ultimately determine the brain's structure, which governs the child's interaction with the environment and, in turn, interactively affects the neuroendocrine and epigenetic systems and gene expression (Gudsnuk & Champagne, 2012; McLaughlin, Sheridan, & Lambert, 2014; Fiori & Turecki, 2016). While considering specific contributing factors into the formation of DTD in IAPI children, we should constantly keep in mind the interactive and cumulative nature of these factors.

Inherited Transgenerational Trauma as a Factor in DTD Formation

Who are the biological parents of IAPI children? I had the rare opportunity to study legal and medical documentation of children adopted from many countries and brought to my office for an initial assessment. One thing is certain for me: a heartbreaking story about a nice, healthy, young female university student who got pregnant unexpectedly and had to give her child up for adoption because she wanted to continue her studies or did not have the means to support the child belongs completely to the category of urban legends. The inspection of many dozens of adoption court documents presented a collective portrait of destitute, battered, often homeless, unemployed, drug and alcohol addicted women, frequently having several children from different men; some gave birth in jails or drug/alcohol rehabilitation centers or in local hospitals during their rootless roaming from place to place. These women belonged to the lowest social-economic stratum of their societies. Typically, neither prenatal nor postnatal medical attention was available to these mothers and their newly born babies. Poor nutrition, smoking, alcohol and/or drug abuse, exposure to environmental toxins, constant stress, and ongoing social rejection and humiliation are typical characteristics of this population. And the effect of these factors does not end with them.

Prenatal stress in mothers of IAPI children forms the biological foundation of intergenerational trauma. Human epidemiology studies suggest that deviant development in parental generations caused by nutritional deficit, chemical infusion, and psychological stressors can be passed on to children by nongenetic processes. Such nongenetic transmissions of detrimental effects across generations have been considered as causes of human health and behavior problems (Kaufman, Plotsky, Nemeroff, & Chamey, 2000; Meaney, 2001, 2010). An increasing body of research has demonstrated how development is influenced by intrauterine experience: a high level of maternal stress during pregnancy has a negative effect on a child's development (Franklin et al., 2010; Weinberg & Tronick, 1998). An offspring of a traumatized mother inherits a variation of her trauma by virtue of being born by this woman. An example of this intergenerational traumatic transfer is shown in the children of Holocaust survivors, who come to share their parents' trauma-based biochemistry in the absence of having experienced any objective trauma themselves (Yehuda & Siever, 1997; Scharf, 2007). In other words, stress in parents results in epigenetic changes in children.

Based on my study of the legal records for the adopted children from Russia, Ukraine, and other countries of Eastern Europe, I discovered that many of the biological mothers of these children were the "graduates" of orphanages themselves. In addition, in some cases, I have found that the parents of these women also belonged to the same lowest social stratum. This means that during their tragic and usually short life cycles, the grandparents might have passed to their daughters and grandchildren the stress and traumas of their own lives, forming the biological foundation of intergenerational trauma.

The Impact of Early Toxic Stress on the Formation of DTD and the Rigidity of Stress Response

Following the classification of Shonkoff and Garner (2012), stress (a state of mental or emotional strain or tension resulting from adverse or demanding circumstances) can be categorized as positive, helping to guide growth; tolerable, which while not helpful will cause no permanent damage; and toxic—harmful for a person. The evolution prepares humans' CNS to convert manageable doses of stress into adaptation: in typical positive development, stress hormones initiate biological changes that enhance neural plasticity, learning, and adaptive coping responses (Huether, 1998). Toxic stress, however, overcomes the child's immature coping mechanisms and lead to long-term impairments. As formulated by Cozolino (2014, p. 258), *"extreme and prolonged stress to a young child's CNS fundamentally overwhelms this child's capacity to stimulate neural circuits to grow, to shape sensory-motor functioning, and to help regulate the autonomic nervous system."*

The subjective nature of stress should be emphasized: what causes a traumatic impact on one child may not produce the same effect on another. The reaction to the potentially trauma-produced event(s) or condition(s) is predetermined by the child's genetic equipment, system of social support, previous trauma history, and many other factors. When the stress is "toxic" (that is, extremely adverse), repetitive, and severe, and social/emotional buffering is absent or insufficient, like in the case of abandoned and motherless children, then traumatic alterations may result in epigenetic modifications, changes in brain structure and function, and in the formation of behavior patterns that may be maladaptive in many contexts. It is, obviously, a contributing factor to the later psychosocial problems with emotional regulation, impulse control, logical thinking, and social behavior seen in maltreated children (Putnam, 2006).

The stress response, while essential in times of threat, is designed to return to a baseline state when the threat is no longer present: this is a typical pattern of normal human functioning (Gunnar, 1998). But we do not see that in many international adoptees: adversity in early life shapes the experience-dependent maturation of stress-regulating pathways underlying emotional functions. Practitioners working with the IAPI population observed that children who experienced traumatic events in the past continue to experience heightened neurochemical reactions in the present without the existence of a threat (Gunnar & Donzella, 2002; De Bellis, Hooper, Spratt, & Woolley, 2009; Pollak et al., 2010). The release of adrenaline facilitates the reinforcement of threat memory, and there is some evidence that failure to regulate the sympathetic nervous system response may lead to stronger encoding of a traumatic memory (Heim & Nemeroff, 2002; Heim & Binder, 2012).

Neglect as an Extreme Toxic Stress: The Relational Nature of DTD in IAPI Children

IAPI children's adverse experiences come in many shapes and forms, and, as yet, neglect has emerged as the most devastating cause of DTD. Neglect of a child, expressed in a lack of stimulation and physical and emotional support, is more detrimental to development than other adverse childhood experiences. Infants are totally dependent on their caregivers, and they experience extreme distress when neglected. An almost total stimulus deprivation of infants can lead to developmental delays, depression, and even death, and the lesser degrees of neglect have been associated with a number of social and mental health impairments (Schore, 2003; Eisenberger, Taylor, Gable, Hilmert, & Leiberman, 2007). According to van der Kolk, neglected infants and children develop disorganized/disoriented attachment relationships, which are expressed as an unpredictable approach-and-avoidance pattern toward caregivers, the inability to accept comfort from caregivers, rage directed at attachment figures, and pathological self-regulatory behaviors (van der Kolk, 2003, 2005, 2015).

Neglect has stable detrimental characteristics: it is prolonged (chronic); it is interpersonal; it has an early life onset (Hildyard & Wolfe, 2002; Champagne, 2010; Dudley, Li, Kobor, Kippin, & Bredy, 2011). The most damaging form of neglect is total abandonment, which damages the very core of human nature—social connectedness. Through the history of human evolution, total abandonment results in the death of a young child (Baumeister & Leary, 1995). As noted by Cozolino (2014, pp. 295–296),

> *Given that the brain is both a social organ and an organ of adaptation, a lack of stimulation results in the abnormal development of experience-dependent structures, such as the cerebral cortex, corpus callosum, and hippocampus. These abnormalities are likely the result of the negative effects of chronically high levels of stress hormones combined with inadequate emotional regulation, required by the developing social brain.*

A good deal of research defines traumatic experiences in two major groups: non-interpersonal (such as natural disasters or technological catastrophes) and interpersonal experiences, such as neglect, abandonment, sexual/physical abuse, life in an institution, and chronic exposure to overt hostility. It was commonly agreed that trauma of an interpersonal nature has more severe and lasting consequences (Schore, 2003; Hibbard, Barlow, & Macmillan, 2012; Cozolino, 2014). In interpersonal trauma, the severity increases with the closeness of the relationship. Thus, abandonment or violence inflicted by the mother would be experienced by a child as extremely devastating. As Cozolino (2014, p. 280) writes,

> *The most damaging element of early complex trauma is in an approach/avoidance conflict. If a child needs to feel connected in order to heal but is too afraid to trust because he/she can become fearful and dysregulated in relationships, the child is stuck in the trap.*

From the remedial and therapeutic perspective, it is important to realize that neglect, as the extreme form of toxic stress, fundamentally affects what Bowlby (1980) called an "internal working model"—a mental representation of our relationships with our primary caregivers that becomes a template for future relationships and allows individuals to predict, control, and manipulate their environment. In a typical development, this "internal model" is the result of nurturing interaction with a caregiver. If such an interaction is absent, as in abandonment, or distorted, as in a dysfunctional family or institution, the long-term development of the "internal working model" is compromised. One of the most significant consequences of DTD in IAPI children is the formation of the "internal model" of the surroundings as an unsafe and unpredictable place to live, which in turn shapes the related "survival" mode of behavior.

An extension to Bowlby's "internal working model" is Cozolino's "internalized mother" concept. If a child is abandoned at birth or within the first months of life, he or she does not have a chance to develop a very special experience, which Cozolino calls an "internal mother" (2014, pp. 116–117):

> *Early in life, we learn the smells, sights, touch, and sounds of our mother's presence, unconsciously associating these experiences with our bodily and emotional states. We all have what has been called an internalized mother, a network of visceral, somatic, and emotional memories of our interactions with our mothers, which are thought to serve as the core of self-esteem, our ability to self-soothe, and the foundation of our adult relationships. This early, preverbal dyad establishes the biological, behavioral, and psychological structure of our expectations about other people, the world, and the future.*

A close relationship between the quality of early life and mental health in later life is a proven scientific fact. Over the years, it has frequently been suggested that the lack of "mothering," appropriate social/emotional experiences, and relationships with a few consistent caregivers are the primary causes of developmental delays and deficiencies in IAPI children (Rutter, 2000). While most of the early studies were on children residing in orphanages—who were deficient in almost every dimension—even children who are reared in relatively good orphanages but are subject to social and emotional neglect display many of trauma-related characteristics (St. Petersburg—USA Orphanage Research Team, 2009).

The Issue of Comorbidity and Misdiagnosing of IAPI Children

The issue of coexistence of two or more different diseases (comorbidity) has major practical implications in the context of rehabilitation and remediation of IAPI children. The specific mental health disorder and DTD can be separate issues, each with an independent course, yet each able to influence the properties of the other. Symptoms of trauma include patterns of many other mental health disorders, which often leads to misdiagnosing children having DTD with another disorder. The most outstanding case in the field of international adoption is, of course, so-called institutional autism, when IAPI children with learned post-orphanage, trauma-produced behaviors present a number of "autistic-like" features and based on that are misdiagnosed as children with autism spectrum disorder condition (see more on this topic in Chapter 6).

Adopted children who, due to DTD, are constantly aroused and hypervigilant to real or imagined adverse events or conditions may be easily diagnosed with attention-deficit/hyperactivity disorder (ADHD) (see a detailed discussion in Chapter 6). Youngsters who are unresponsive, avoidant, and withdrawn as a consequence of DTD may be diagnosed as depressed. Those who are conditioned by DTD to acting out or presenting "proactive" (not provoked) aggressive behaviors may be mistakenly recognized as having oppositional defiant disorder. However, for children who have been experiencing a prolonged traumatization in early childhood, "acting out" behaviors, a lack of empathy, and self-centeredness can be the consequences of trauma and deeply embedded survival skills. As a result, many IAPI children are given a range of diagnoses that are missing the underlying general cause of their conditions, thus subjecting these children to maltreatment. As stated by D'Andrea et al. (2012, p. 7), due to a range of psychiatric symptoms found in traumatized children, *"multiple comorbid diagnoses are necessary—but not necessarily accurate—to describe many victimized children, potentially leading to both undertreatment and overtreatment."*

The most complicated is interconnectedness between DTD and PTSD in IAPI children. There is a distinct difference between these two conditions, which is described in detail in Chapter 6. There are also a number of common presentations in overt behavior. In understanding the differences between PTSD and DTD, it is necessary to realize that a child afflicted with DTD may still have symptoms and even the full-blown condition of PTSD.

Young children who have been traumatized multiple times often experience developmental delays across a broad spectrum, including cognitive, language, motor, and socialization skills; they tend to display multiple disturbances with various presentations, thus meeting numerous clinical diagnoses. And yet each of these diagnoses captures only a limited aspect of the traumatized child, while a more comprehensive view of the impact of complex trauma provides a focused developmental approach.

In terms of symptomatic presentation of DTD in IAPI children, the notion of interconnectedness of physiological and psychological aspects has vital significance for the proper understanding of psychosomatic manifestations of the presence of DTD, as seen from the clinical case of George, an 8-year-old boy.

Clinical Case: George, a Pseudo-Autistic Boy

George was adopted just before his fourth birthday from an orphanage in Ethiopia. While in the custody of his young and single biological mother for the first 20 months of his life, George was subjected to unhealthy living conditions. George's adoptive parents listed such traumatic events in George's pre-adoption life as abandonment, severe malnourishment, deprivation of basic conditions for growth and development, exposure to toxic substances (heavy metals), and a two-year-long placement in a state-run institution with dismal conditions. When I saw him at the age of 8 years old, George had come a long way from being a malnourished, weak child to become a physically healthy boy with no medical restrictions for any age-appropriate activities or a need for mandatory medical follow-ups.

From the very beginning of his life in his adoptive family, his parents were concerned about consistent patterns of George's behavior at home, such as aggressiveness against his parents and siblings, poor self-regulation of emotions and conduct, impulsivity, temper tantrums resulting in property destruction, somewhat bizarre behavior like licking door knobs, biting his mother's hands, and touching the private parts of both his mother and father.

At the age of 6, he was diagnosed by a local child psychiatrist with "autism," but with a modifier: "atypical." As the parents reported, one more mental health professional agreed with the diagnosis, another rejected it outright. In desperation, the adoptive parents brought George to our office, wanting to know whether George's social/emotional functioning had been determined by his early childhood deprivations or whether it was a genuine neurological impairment and psychiatric disorder (autism).

Initially, I reviewed about 70 minutes of video files of home-based behavior of the child prepared by the parents. The following patterns of behavior were noted:

- Extreme motor dysregulation: at times chaotic and at times repetitive movements. George appeared restless and agitated in the highest degree: he was jumping, running, and spinning around, as if there was an overwhelming, uncontrollable urge to move to discharge tension. In some episodes, he appeared to be on edge of complete disengagement from reality; in other episodes, these appeared to be controlled, planned, and goal-directed movements.
- Intense verbal restlessness: "baby-talk"—repeating phrases, poorly articulated sounded-out words, bizarre screaming (similar to what one can observe in children afflicted with autism), but no echolalia. On the other hand, the same child spoke absolutely normally for a long time, with grammatically correct sentences, proper pronunciation of sounds, and age-appropriate word usage.
- Oppositional, defiant behavior in response to parents' instructions and demands: obvious patterns of challenging, provoking behavior, and destroying or damaging property and house items in front of parents. The parents' words and calm tone had no effect on George as if the boy kept testing the boundaries of his parents' patience.
- Some bizarre behaviors: George was smiling, giggling, and loudly laughing while performing disturbing, defiant, and oppositional

acts. He threw his body against the wall or on the floor, dropped his pants and danced, and he often rocked back and forth.

- Sensory integration issues: the boy definitely was unable to processes sensory inputs in a purposeful and organized manner. The observed reactions to touch, movement, and visual/auditory stimuli were way different from developmental expectations for George's age: both under- and over-responsiveness and extreme sensory-seeking actions, were noticeable.

In general, a combination of an extremely dysregulated CNS and signs of pervasive developmental disorder (an atypical autism) could be suggested based on the video recording submitted by the parents.

During the interviews (and through many e-mail messages) with George's parents and two of his teachers, I found the following:

George routinely exhibited aggressive, violent behavior toward his family members with no sign of remorse and no empathy. However, this violent and aggressive behavior was not reported in school or observed outside of the house. His parents did not see any obvious triggers of his behavior: it appeared suddenly and was not visibly related to what was going on. It appeared that George saw entertainment in forcing all family members to keep him from accidentally hurting himself or deliberately hurting others. The most distressing for his parents was that George's violence was never accompanied by any signs of anger or distress; instead, he laughed and seemed delighted with the result. George's parents recognized that George did not receive empathy during the first four years of his life, and perhaps empathy had to be received to be learned.

At home, George often experienced deep-rooted tension that, in his parents' words, "appeared suddenly and out of the blue." When his tension mounted and his ability to refrain from outbursts diminished, George released tension through physical agitation that might take the form of physical or verbal acting out behavior. Inner tension is a feeling of nervousness and acute mood discomfort. This drive makes purposeless actions practically unavoidable, almost compulsory for him. A bystander would find it impossible to empathize or even understand the tension that forces a child to act with intense rage. However, for George, these actions led to inner relief in spite of making his life, objectively, less positive and, at times, dismal (rejection, punishment, reprimands, deprivation of acceptance, etc.). He might well recognize that these were not acceptable behaviors, but he had no control and could not prevent them on his own. It's important to realize that this behavior does not have purpose and does not have "triggers." It has an inner dynamic, dictated by the child's nervous system and is relatively free from environmental influences. It may start "out of the blue," and it may disappear suddenly.

George often raged when his meal was placed in front of him. He viewed the quantity offered as too small—even when the amount was far too much for him to actually eat. George behaved this way from the early days when he was first brought home. This is an understandable reaction for anyone like George who has suffered severe malnutrition and horrific neglect during the first four years of his life. George's parents repeatedly reassured him that once he finished what was offered, he could always have more. George eventually calmed down and ate, then continued calming the more he ate.

School-related issues: George had been in a special education self-contained small class for the last two years with the educational classification "other health impaired." School-based testing found him functioning in the average range of cognitive abilities and academically about a year below his current grade placement. In school, he did not exhibit the aggressive behaviors, but was impulsive, restless, and inattentive with occasional inappropriate behaviors, such as pulling down his pants for the entertainment of his classmates. As observed by his teachers, George could be a composed and obedient child until suddenly he experienced fear, anxiety, and an urge for an emotional outburst. The teachers could not explain the triggers for such behavior. George's reactions to social events, interpersonal relationships, and overall adaptive behavior could be different every day. In his teachers' opinion, George was more vulnerable to change in daily routine, more prone to frustration related to classroom assignments, and less capable of self-regulating his goal-directed behavior than were his classmates, even in his special education class.

George indeed at times demonstrates some patterns of behavior that are similar to those typical to children with an autism spectrum disorder (ASD). However, on other occasions, he appeared as "normal" as his classmates. It was my conclusion that his "autistic-like" patterns of behavior are different in etiology (but at times similar in presentation) from typical ASD children and produced by complex childhood trauma and learned "institutional" behavior. This is not an unusual case in internationally adopted post-institutionalized children (Gindis, 2008).

George continuously demonstrated a markedly disturbed and developmentally inappropriate social relatedness with parents and siblings. He demonstrated the presence of a psychiatric condition known as attachment disorder (AD) that encompasses a wide range of symptoms of varying magnitudes, particularly in the social/behavioral area. The etiology of this disorder is complex, but early childhood deprivation and institutionalization are definitely a part of it. AD is a "continuum" disorder with a wide variety of symptoms. George has a severe variation of AD, with most behavioral characteristics clearly presented, thus predisposing this child to experience significant difficulties in forming age-appropriate and culturally approved relationships with significant others (his parents first of all).

Typical features of the emotional makeup of a post-institutionalized child with DTD are "hyper-arousal" and/or "dissociation/depression" (a separation of emotions resulting in inadequate social interaction, lacking empathy and understanding of a cause/effect relationship). As defined by B. Perry et al. (1995, p. 279), repetitive traumatization of a child leads to

> *a sensitized neural response resulting from a specific pattern of repetitive neural activation due to repetitive traumatizing experiences. Sensitization occurs when this pattern of activation results in an altered, more sensitive system. Once sensitized, the same neural activity can be elicited by less intense external stimuli.*

Traumatic events in early childhood have the capacity to "redefine" the baseline level of the CNS involved in the stress response.

Inner deep-seated trauma inhibits George's ability to respond meaningfully to relationships with adults and peers. George's conditions are to be addressed by a complex set of actions that should include medical monitoring (to take care of impulsivity and restlessness), parental counseling (to manage home-based behavior), and trauma-informed cognitive/behavioral therapy, individual and family, provided by a therapist experienced in working with IAPI children.

Symptomatic Presentation of DTD in IAPI Children

Physiological Symptoms of DTD

Physiological symptoms of DTD, as described in research literature, include sensory integration difficulties, musculoskeletal pain, abnormally decreased or increased pain threshold, sleep disturbance, hyper-arousal and hypo-arousal, problems with digestion, oversensitivity to touch or sound, and other physiological indications (Carlson & Earls, 1997; Cook et al., 2005; Van der Kolk, 2015). It is a consistent finding that even after years in an adoptive family, IAPI children may continue to demonstrate an abnormal response to stress, both on a basic biological level, such as increased cortisol in salvia (Gunnar & Quevedo, 2007), increased heart rate, and blood pressure (Van der Kolk, 2003; Fisher, 2014), and in observable behavior. Physiological symptoms of DTD are most comprehensively presented in a number of monographs, authored by B. Rothschild (2000), P. Ogden et al. (2006), S. Fisher (2014), and B. van der Kolk (2015), to cite just a few relevant major publications that allow me to concentrate on the psychological symptomatology of DTD in IAPI children.

Psychological Symptomatology of DTD in IAPI Children

Dysregulated High Psychological Functions

Psychological symptomatology of DTD in IAPI children is multifaceted, but the most prominent feature is the grossly dysregulated high psychological functions: poorly modulated emotions, disorganized cognition, disrupted attention, weakly controlled behavior. Dysregulation of affect and behavior may be manifested in both externalized (as described in George's case) and internalized symptoms, such as depression, anxieties, phobias, and eating disorders (Rogosch & Cicchetti, 2005; Cloitre, 2005; Ford, Vostanis, Meltzer, & Goodman, 2007). Van der Kolk (2003, 2005, p. 215) defines psychological symptoms of DTD as an inability to concentrate and pay attention; chronic anger, fear, and anxiety; self-loathing and self-destructive behavior; limitations in the self-regulation of feelings and behavior; aggression against others; dissociation; and an incapacity to negotiate satisfactory interpersonal relationships.

Self-regulation of emotions includes the accurate identification of internal emotional states and the selection of a socially acceptable way of external expression of emotions. Many IAPI children exhibit impairment on both stages. Conversely, some IAPI children may respond with the general numbing of their emotions, "shutting them down," and lack responsiveness to the external world (Tarren-Sweeney, 2008). Dysregulated emotional, cognitive and language functioning is considered in more details in Chapters 4, 5, and 6 of this book).

Distorted "Internal Working Model"

Second in rank in the catalogue of DTD symptomatology in IAPI children, I would put the children's distorted perception of the world and themselves, a malformed "internal working model," as it was called by Bowlby (1980). In a typical development, internal working model is a secure base from which to explore the social and physical world, as it results from the nurturing interactions with the caregiver. This "internal working model" is a cognitive framework, encompassing mental representations for understanding the world, the self, and others. As stated by Bowlby and others (e.g., Cozolino, 2014), the internal working model is defined by the children's internalization of the emotional and cognitive properties of their social relationships with prime caregivers in early childhood. The early caregiver relationship has a profound impact on a child's development of a coherent sense of self. Responsive, sensitive caretaking and positive early life experiences allow a child to develop a model of self as generally worthy and competent. In contrast, repetitive experiences of harm or rejection by significant others and the associated failure to develop age-appropriate competencies are likely to lead to a sense of one's self as ineffective, helpless, deficient, and unlovable. The child's self-perception and worldviews get distorted by rejection, violence, hostility, and fear.

Indeed, IAPI children assemble their internal working model in a manner that depicts the world as a dangerous place to live and themselves as unwanted and dreadful, deserving only continued traumatic experiences. Children who perceive themselves as powerless or incompetent and who expect others to reject and despise them are more likely to blame themselves for negative experiences and have problems eliciting and responding to social support. Therapists working with IAPI children agree that these children are more resistant to talking about internal states, particularly their negative feelings. Lowered estimates of self-competence are already seen during the pre-adolescent time; by adolescence, they tend to suffer from a high degree of self-blame (Teicher et al., 2003; van der Kolk, 2003; Sonuga-Barke, Schlotz, & Kreppner, 2010; McLean, 2016).

State of Hyper-Arousal and Hypo-Arousal (Dissociation)

These two opposite states of the CNS can be found in same IAPI child at different times. Specifically, hyper-arousal presents itself in excessive vigilance, agitation, irritability, constant state of rage, and "proactive" aggression, while hypo-arousal is evident in withdrawal and disengagement. In the dissociated state, emotions, sensations, perception, and thought are broken into separate fragments and are not processed coherently. Dissociation is a defense against fear or pain; it allows children to escape mentally from frightening or painful things that are happening to them.

Each of these response patterns activate a unique combination of neural systems, literally blocking the adequate processing of what is happening in social relations, in the classroom, or in self-perception. Chronic trauma exposure may lead to an over-reliance on hyper-arousal or dissociation (in my clinical experience—very often in the same child) as a coping mechanism that, in turn, can exacerbate difficulties with behavioral management and affect regulation and self-concept (Belsky, Bakermans-Kranenburg, & Van IJzendoorn, 2007; Heim & Binder, 2012; Larkin, Felitti, & Anda, 2014).

Although there is consensus that early stress leads to an ongoing dysregulation of the CNS stress response system (McEwen, 2012), the exact nature of this dysregulation is debated (McCrory et al., 2010). The research findings suggest that the stress response system can either become chronically overactivated or under-responsive over time (McEwen, 2012; McLaughlin et al., 2014; McCrory, Gerin, & Viding, 2017) in response to a variety of factors (e.g., severity, chronicity, and timing of trauma) that are currently unclear. Therefore, while the findings support the idea that childhood trauma is associated with a disruption in stress sensitivity and response, they do not uniformly support the idea of chronic hyper-activation, as suggested by some researchers (e.g., Perry, 2006).

The rigidity of internalized traumatic consequences is astonishing in IAPI children. The templates of survival behavior, adaptive for an objectively adverse situation of dysfunctional family and institution, become maladaptive once the child is in the objectively favorable situation with the adoptive family. To the great surprise and frustration of adoptive parents, an international adoptee reacts as if he or she is still in an adverse situation of stress and danger. Traumatic memories are stored in the more "primitive" areas of the brain, so they are less accessible to language, logic, and reasoning. This may impede adequate responses and lead the child to regression to earlier developmental stages. At the same time, limited language and undifferentiated memories of emotional strain may lower a child's capacity to relieve the pain through verbalization, resulting in tantrums and acting out. In many IAPI children, the traumatic experience remains at the same intensity level for many years, leading to constant emotional tension (Marinus & Juffer, 2011; Benjet et al., 2011).

Difficulties in Forming and Sustaining Social Connectedness

The fourth in the ranking of prominent traits of DTD in IAPI children is difficulty forming social connectedness. DTD powerfully interferes with the formation of interpersonal relatedness. As I mentioned earlier, IAPI children have difficulty accurately reading social cues and social demands of ongoing situations. Further, they are often out of tune with others, either socially withdrawn or aggressive to other children and family members. Unable to regulate their emotions, they tend to scare other children away and lack reliable playmates and chums. Traumatized children often have difficulty learning collaborative play and reciprocal relationships with others. Difficulties in forming and sustaining social connections are discussed in Chapter 6 of this book.

In addition to the earlier reviewed symptoms of DTD in IAPI children, there is a range of specific psychological symptoms of DTD that are found only in this population: an abrupt first-language attrition, cumulative cognitive deficit, and post-orphanage behavior. These specific features will be discussed in the next chapters of this book.

Resilience to the Consequences of DTD in IAPI Children

Resiliency is the ability to cope with life stresses. As a theoretical construct, resilience is defined in various ways but, essentially, it refers to a dynamic process of forbearance leading to positive adaptation in the face of significant adversity (Luthar, Cicchetti, & Becker, 2000; Calhoun & Tedeschi, 2006). It implies that the impairment and suffering that follow trauma do not preclude concurrently restorative and successful adjustment, which results in positive development (Bonanno, 2004; Layne, Warren, Watson, & Shalev, 2007). Moreover, adverse childhood experience in some children becomes the source of strength and creativity, as known from the biographies of many famous individuals. "What does not kill us makes us stronger," as Friedrich Nietzsche said. Why do some orphanage residents carry the deep scars of institutional rearing for life, while the others, for all practical purposes, successfully mix in with the general population? What causes a different outcome after the same traumatic experience? Why do IAPI children have DTD in different degrees? Why do they react differently to the adversity of early childhood and post-adoption stress? All my professional life, I was fascinated by those mysterious sources of resilience in IAPI children, whether they are rooted in individual neurological differences, social/emotional support, or learned social skills. Our understanding of the psychological nature of resilience in IAPI children may have, potentially, the most significant benefits for therapeutic practice and educational remediation. The variability of outcomes of post-adoption upbringing in children who had similar pre-adoption experiences is so remarkable that we need to know what constitutes resilience alongside specific vulnerabilities in IAPI children.

Based on my clinical experience, I suggest, for further discussion, the following factors that in my opinion have shown links to IAPI children's resilience to the consequences of DTD:

1. Social connectedness: if an IAPI child is lucky to have in his or her pre-adoptive and post-adoptive life a person available for productive intimate social/emotional interactions, or the child is predisposed by his or her individual nature to form and maintain such social relationships, then the chances of effective resilience for an IAPI child could be increased significantly. The greatest threat to resilience is the breakdown of external protective systems.

2. Individual characteristics of a child: temperament (easygoing personality, innate positive disposition, and sociable demeanor) and certain personality traits (positive beliefs about oneself, motivation to learn copying strategies, etc.)

3. A specific gift in any domains (art, sport, craftsmanship, etc.) may be a key to overcoming the consequences of DTD and even physical/neurological disability. Just one example: Oksana Masters, a member of the U.S. Paralympics team, the eight-time Paralympics medalist, was adopted from a Ukrainian orphanage as a physically handicapped child at the age of 6 (the article from *NY Times*, March 9, 2018: "Oksana Masters Road From a Ukrainian Orphanage to Paralympic Stardom"[6]). Those adoptive parents, who were able to discover or to develop a special ability in their kids and reinforce it by their

endless scaffolding and encouragement, led the children to an accomplishment and related self-confidence that had surmounted the DTD.

4. Time: length of exposure and severity of toxic stress. One factor, used as an explanation for positive outcome of adoption, has been mentioned consistently in research and throughout this book: the age of adoption. The research data and clinical experience clearly indicate that developmental catchups and developmental improvements are greater when children transition to their adoptive families at a young age, preferably before the second birthday (Ford et al., 2007; Hibbard et al., 2012; Compton, 2016). However, the relationship between resilience and age of adoption is not as direct as it appears: the age of adoption factor is mediated by several other variables (e.g., the severity of the pre-orphanage and orphanage experience). As research shows, the DTD effects may well be observed after as little as six months, in some cases, and within the first two years for many cases (Sonuga-Barke, 2010).

As of today, the bottom line is that we know too little about the nature of resilience in IAPI children, despite the practical significance of this issue.

To conclude, in relation to IAPI children, the notion of developmental trauma disorder, relational in nature and often on the background of birth-related neurological weaknesses, is the most productive explanatory paradigm. Indeed, DTD consistently mediates the development of IAPI children. The acceptance of this concept allows us to determine the underlying causes of many issues in IAPI children and to understand their neurophysiological and psychological symptomatic presentations better. DTD in IAPI children differs in many aspects from what we observe in the general population of children affected by adverse childhood experiences. In the IAPI population, DTD comes as the synergetic effect of weakened neurology, epigenetic, and transgenerational trauma, overwhelming pre-adoption stress, and the ordeal of culture and language adjustment after the adoption.

Notes

1. http://apps.who.int/iris/bitstream/handle/10665/43943/9789241563703_eng.pdf;sequence=1
2. www.orphandoctor.com/services/assessment/russian.html
3. www.adoptmed.org/topics/glossary-of-russian-medical-terms.html
4. www.cdc.gov/nchs/slaits/nsch.htm
5. www.childtrends.org/publications/prevalence-adverse-childhood-experiences-nationally-state-race-ethnicity/
6. https://www.nytimes.com/2018/03/09/sports/paralympics-oksana-masters.html

References

Barclay, L. (2005). Extreme prematurity linked to cognitive impairment at school age. *New England Journal of Medicine, 352,* 9–19.

Baumeister, R. F., & Leary, M. R. (1995). The need to belong: Desire for interpersonal attachments as a fundamental human motivation. *Psychological Bulletin, 117,* 497–529.

Belsky, J., Bakermans-Kranenburg, M., & Van IJzendoorn, M. (2007). For better and for worse: Differential susceptibility to environmental influences. *Current Directions in Psychological Science, 16,* 300–304.

Benjet, C., Borges, G., Mendez, E., Fleiz, C., & Medina-Mora, M. (2011). The association of chronic adversity with psychiatric disorder and disorder severity in adolescents. *European Child & Adolescent Psychiatry, 20,* 459–468.

Bonanno, G. A. (2004). Loss, trauma, and human resilience. *American Psychologist, 59,* 20–28.

Bowlby, J. (1980). *Attachment and loss* (Vol. 3). New York, NY: Basic Books.

Calhoun, L. G., & Tedeschi, R. G. (2006). *Handbook of posttraumatic growth: Research and practice.* New York, NY: Lawrence Erlbaum Associates.

Carlson, M., & Earls, F. (1997). Psychological and neuroendocrinological sequala of early social deprivation in institutionalized children in Romania. *Annals of N Y Academy of Science, 807,* 419–428.

Champagne, F. A. (2010). Epigenetic influence of social experiences across the lifespan. *Developmental Psychobiology, 52,* 299–311.

Cloitre, M. (2005). Beyond PTSD: Emotion regulation and interpersonal problems as predictors of functional impairment in survivors of childhood abuse. *Behavior Therapy, 36,* 119–124.

Compton, R. (2016). Adoption beyond borders. How international adoption benefit children. Oxford U. Press, New York, USA.

Cook, A., Spinazzola, J., Ford, J., Lanktree, C., Blaustein, M., Cloitre, M., . . . van der Kolk, B. (2005). Complex trauma in children and adolescents. *Psychiatric Annals, 35*(5), 390–398.

Cozolino, L. (2014). *The Neuroscience of human relationships: Attachment and the developing social brain* (2nd ed.). New York: W.W. Norton and Co.

D'Andrea, W., Ford, J., Stolbach, B., Spinazzola, J., & van der Kolk, B. (2012). Understanding interpersonal trauma in children: Why we need a developmentally appropriate trauma diagnosis. *American Journal of Orthopsychiatry, 82*(2), 187–200.

De Bellis, M. D., Hooper, S. R., Spratt, E. G., & Woolley, D. P. (2009). Neuropsychological findings in childhood neglect and their relationships to pediatric PTSD. *Journal of the International Neuropsychological Society, 15,* 868–878.

Diagnostic and statistical manual of mental disorders, 5th ed. (DSM-5). (2013) Washington, DC: American Psychiatric Association.

Dudley, K., Li, X., Kobor, M., Kippin, T., & Bredy, T. (2011). Epigenetic mechanisms mediating vulnerability and resilience to psychiatric disorders. *Neuroscience Biobehavioral Review, 35*(7), 1544–1551.

Eisenberger, N., Taylor, S., Gable, S., Hilmert, C., & Leiberman, M. (2007). Neural pathways link social support to attenuated neuroendocrine stress responses. *Neuroimage, 5*(4), 1601–1612.

Fiori, L., & Turecki, G. (2016). Investigating epigenetic consequences of early-life adversity: some methodological considerations. *European Journal of Psychotraumatology*, 7(10). Retrieved November 8, 2016, from www.ncbi. nlm.nih.gov/pmc/articles/PMC5106862/

Fisher, S. (2014). *Neurofeedback in the treatment of developmental trauma*. New York: Norton.

Ford, T., Vostanis, P., Meltzer, H., & Goodman, R. (2007). Psychiatric disorder among British children looked after by local authorities: Comparison with children living in private households. *British Journal of Psychiatry*, *190*, 319–325.

Franklin, T. B., Russig, H., Weiss, I. C., Graff, J., Linder, N., Michalon, A., . . . Mansuy, I. M. (2010). Epigenetic transmission of the impact of early stress across generations. *Biological Psychiatry*, *68*, 408–415.

Gindis, B. (2008). Institutional autism in children adopted internationally: Myth or reality? *International Journal of Special Education*, *23*(3), 124–129).

Gudsnuk, K., & Champagne, F. (2012). Epigenetic influence of stress and the social environment. *Institute of Laboratory Animal Resources (ILAR) Journal*, *53*(3–4), 279–288. Retrieved from www.ncbi.nlm.nih.gov/pmc/articles/ PMC4021821/

Gunnar, M. R. (1998). Quality of care and buffering of neuroendocrine stress reactions: Potential effects on the developing human brain. *Preventive Medicine*, 27, 208–211.

Gunnar, M. R., & Donzella, B. (2002). Social regulation of cortisol level in early human development. *Psychoneuroendocrinology*, 27, 199–220.

Gunnar, M. R., & Quevedo, K. (2007). The neurobiology of stress and development. *Annual Review of Psychology*, *58*, 145–173.

Heim, C., & Binder, E. (2012). Current research trends in early life stress and depression: Review of human studies on sensitive periods, gene: Environment interactions, and epigenetics. *Experimental Neurology*, *233*(1), 102–111.

Heim, C., & Nemeroff, C. B. (2002). Neurobiology of early life stress: Clinical studies. *Seminars in Clinical Neuropsychiatry*, 7, 147–159.

Hibbard, R., Barlow, J., & Macmillan, H. (2012). Psychological maltreatment. *Pediatrics*, *130*(2), 372–378. Retrieved from http://pediatrics.aappublications. org/content/130/2/372

Hildyard, K. L., & Wolfe, D. A. (2002). Child neglect: Developmental issues and outcomes. *Child Abuse and Neglect*, *26*, 679–695.

Huether, C. (1998). Stress and the adaptive self-organization of neuronal connectivity during early childhood. *International Journal of Developmental Neuroscience*, *16*, 297–306.

Kaufman, J., Plotsky, P., Nemeroff, C., & Chamey, D. (2000). Effects of early adverse experiences on brain structure and function: Clinical implications. *Biological Psychiatry*, *48*, 778–790.

Larkin, H., Felitti, V., & Anda, R. (2014). Social work and adverse childhood experiences research: Implications for practice and health policy. *Social Work in Public Health*, *29*(1), 1–16.

Layne, C. M., Warren, J. S., Watson, P. J., & Shalev, A. Y. (2007). Risk, vulnerability, resistance, and resilience: Toward an integrative conceptualization of posttraumatic adaptation. In M. J. Friedman, T. M. Keane, & P. A. Resick (Eds.), *Handbook of PTSD: Science and practice* (pp. 497–520). New York: Guilford Press.

Luthar, S. S., Cicchetti, D., & Becker, B. (2000). The construct of resilience: A critical evaluation and guidelines for future work. *Child Development, 71,* 543–562.

Marinus, H., & Juffer, M. (2011). Children in institutional care: Delayed development and resilience. *Monographs of the Society for Research in Child Development, 76*(4), 8–30.

Marmot, M., & Wilkinson, R. G. (Eds.). (1999). *Social determinants of health.* Oxford, UK: Oxford University Press.

Mather, M., Bridgewater, N., Way, J., & Haworth, G. (2017). The quality of medical information given to prospective intercountry adopters in England. *Adoption & Fostering, 41*(1), 52–61.

McCrory, E., De Brito, S. A., & Viding, E. (2010). Research review: The neurobiology and genetics of maltreatment and adversity. *Journal Child Psychology and Psychiatry, 51,* 1079–1095.

McCrory, E., Gerin, M., & Viding, E. (2017). Annual research review: Childhood maltreatment, latent vulnerability and the shift to preventative psychiatry: The contribution of functional brain imaging. *The Journal of Child Psychology and Psychiatry, 58*(4), 338–357.

McEwen, B. S. (2012). Brain on stress: How the social environment gets under the skin. *Proceedings of the National Academy of Sciences, 109,* 17180–17185.

McLaughlin, K. A., Sheridan, M. A., & Lambert, H. K. (2014). Childhood adversity and neural development: Deprivation and threat as distinct dimensions of early experience. *Neuroscience and Biobehavioural Review, 47,* 578–591.

McLean, S. (2016). The effect of trauma on the brain development of children: Evidence-based principles for supporting the recovery of children in care. *Australian Institute of Family Studies.* Retrieved from https://aifs.gov.au/cfca/publications/effect-trauma-brain-development-children

Meaney, M. (2001). Maternal care, gene expression, and the transmission of individual differences in stress reactivity across generations. *Annual Review in Neuroscience, 24,* 1161–1192.

Meaney, M. (2010). Epigenetics and the biological definition of gene environment interactions. *Child Development, 81,* 41–79.

Mehta, M. A., Golembo, N. I., & Nosarti, C. (2009). Amygdala, hippocampal and corpus callosum size following severe early institutional deprivation: The English and Romanian Adoptees study pilot. *Journal of Child Psychology and Psychiatry, 50*(8), 943–951.

Miller, L. (2005). *The handbook of international adoption medicine: A guide for physicians, parents, and providers.* Oxford, UK: Oxford University Press.

Ogden, P., Minton, K., & Pain, C. (2006). *Trauma and the body: A sensorimotor approach to psychotherapy.* New York: W.W. Norton and Co.

Onis, M., & Yip, R. (1996). The WHO growth chart: Historical considerations and current scientific issues. In M. Porrini & P. Walter (Eds.), *Nutrition in pregnancy and growth* (Vol. 53, pp. 74–89). Basel: Bibliotheka Nutritio et Dieta.

Perry, B. D. (2006). Applying principles of neurodevelopment to clinical work with maltreated and traumatized children: The neurosequential model of therapeutics. In N. B. Webb (Ed.), *Working with traumatized youth in child welfare: Social work practice with children and families* (pp. 27–52). New York: Guilford Press.

Perry, B. D., Pollard, R. A., Blakely, T. L., Baker, W. L., & Vigilante, D. (1995). Childhood trauma, the neurobiology of adaptation, and "use-dependent" development of the brain: How "states" become "traits". *Infant Mental Health Journal, 16*(4), 271–291.

Pollak, S. D., Nelson, C. A., Schlaak, M. F., Roeber, B. J., Wewerka, S. S., Wiik, K. L., . . . Gunnar, M. R. (2010). Neurodevelopmental effects of early deprivation in post-institutionalized children. *Child Development, 81*, 224–236.

Putnam, F. (2006). The impact of trauma on child development. *Juvenile and Family Court Journal, 57*(1), 1–11.

Rodrigues, M., Mello, R., & Fonceca, S. (2006). Learning difficulties in schoolchildren born with very low birth weight. *Journal of Pediatrics, 82*, 6–14.

Rogosch, F., & Cicchetti, D. (2005). Child maltreatment, attention networks, and potential precursors to borderline personality disorder. *Development and Psychopathology, 17*, 1071–1089.

Rothschild, B. (2000). *The body remembers: The psychophysiology of trauma and trauma treatment*. New York: W.W. Norton and Co.

Rutter, M. (2000). Psychosocial influences: Critiques, findings, and research needs. *Development and Psychopathology, 12*, 265–296.

Scharf, M. (2007). Long-term effects of trauma: Psychosocial functioning of the second and third generation of Holocaust survivors. *Development and Psychopathology, 19*, 603–622.

Schore, A. (2003). *Affect regulation and the repair of the self*. New York: W.W. Norton and Co.

Shonkoff, J., & Garner, A. (2012). The lifelong effects of early childhood adversity and toxic stress. *Pediatrics, 129*(1), 232–246.

Sonuga-Barke, E., Schlotz, W., & Kreppner, J. (2010). Differentiation developmental trajectories for conduct, emotion and peer problems following early deprivation. *Monographs of the Society for Research in Child Development, 75*, 102–124.

The St. Petersburg-USA Orphanage Research Team. (2009). The effects of early social-emotional and relationship experience on the development of young orphanage children. *Monographs of the Society for Research in Child Development, 73*(3), vii–295. Publisher: John Wiley & Sons. Contributors Crockenberg, S., Rutter, M., Bakerman-Kranenburg, M., IJzendoorn, M., & Juffer, F.

Tarren-Sweeney, M. (2008). Retrospective and concurrent predictors of the mental health of children in care. *Children and Youth Services Review, 30*, 1–25.

Tedeschi, R. G., & Calhoun, L. G. (2004). Posttraumatic growth: Conceptual foundations and empirical evidence. *Psychological Inquiry, 15*, 1–18.

Teicher, M. H., Andersen, S. L., Polcari, A., Anderson, C. M., Navalta, C. P., & Kim, D. M. (2003). The neurobiological consequences of early stress and childhood maltreatment. *Neuroscience Biobehavior Review, 27*(1–2), 33–44.

Van der Kolk, B. (2003). The neurobiology of childhood trauma and abuse. *Child Adolescent Psychiatric Clinic of North America, 12*, 293–317.

Van der Kolk, B. (2005). Developmental trauma disorder: Towards a rational diagnosis for children with complex trauma history. *Psychiatric Annals, 35*(5), 401–408.

Van der Kolk, B. (2015). *The body keeps the score: Brain, mind, and body in the healing of trauma.* New York: Viking.

Weinberg, M., & Tronick, E. (1998). The impact of maternal psychiatric illness on infant development. *Journal of Clinical Psychiatry, 59,* 53–61.

Weinhold, B., & Weinhold, J. (2015). *Developmental trauma: The game changer in the mental health profession.* Colorado Springs, CO: CIRCLE Press.

Yehuda, R., & Siever, L. (1997). Persistent effect of stress in trauma survivors and their descendants. *Biological Psychiatry, 41,* 1–120.

3 Development Interceded by Trauma in Internationally Adopted Post-Institutionalized Children

Introduction

The notion of child development refers to predominantly irreversible transformations that occur over time as a result of intertwined physical growth, physiological maturation, and social adaptation. There are many different theories of development in contemporary psychology. In this book, the development of IAPI children is considered in the context of Vygotsky's social/cultural theory with its focus on cultural mediation and social connectedness. It is my deepest conviction that this is the most adequate and heuristic theoretical context to discuss a socially induced trauma, complicated by dramatic change of culture and language; it gives the framework for the restoration of higher psychological functions through social relatedness in the new sociocultural environment. Such concepts as "social situation of development," "psychological tools," "direct and mediated learning," "zones of proximal development," the role of language and social context in remediating trauma, and other theoretical postulates are at the core of the theoretical approach of this book.

In Vygotsky's system of thought, a child's development is determined by the interplay of innate biological and social characteristics, with social experience as the central determinant of development (Vygotsky, 1998). After almost a century since his theory was created in the early 1930s, new technologies have revealed a surge of evidence of an early neurophysiological altering of brain structures and functioning under the influence of the social environment (Cozolino, 2014). The understanding that inheritance predisposes a human being to develop in certain ways is undeniable, but social interactions (social connectedness) have a pivotal impact on how these predispositions will be expressed (Champagne et al., 2008; Fox, Levitt, & Nelson, 2010). We now better understand the complex processes of interactions between neurological, endocrine, immune, and metabolic systems and the social environments, specifically interaction with early caregivers. Nurturing relationships lead to the formation of brain pathways that are the prerequisites to age-appropriate behavior, learning, and self-regulation, while neglect, deprivation, and abuse of social relatedness lead to delayed and distorted development (Gunnar & Quevedo, 2007; McCrory, De Brito, & Viding, 2010; Heim & Binder, 2012). Recent research supports Vygotsky's insights that the early social experiences of children become biologically embedded, thus forming the foundation for behavior, cognition, learning, and physical and mental health (McEwan & Gianaros, 2010; Hertzman, 2012; McEwen, 2012; Shonkoff & Garner, 2012). The research points at the early plasticity of brain pathways and the related flexibility in the development of endocrine, immune, and metabolic systems, changing in response to each child's individual social circumstances (Perry, Pollard, Blakely, Baker, & Vigilante, 1995; Nelson, Kendall, & Shields, 2014; Lohmann & Kessels, 2014).

Social Situation of Development in the Life of IAPI Children

The notion of social situation of development (SSD) was constructed by Vygotsky in conjunction with the dynamics of child's development. He wrote (Vygotsky, 1998, Volume 5, p. 198),

> *At the beginning of each age period, there develops a completely original, exclusive, and unique relation, specific to the given age, between the child and the social reality, that surrounds him. We call this relation the social situation of development. . . . It represents the initial moment for all dynamic changes that occur in development during the given period. It determines . . . the path along which the child will acquire ever newer personality characteristics, drawing them from the social reality as the basic source of development, the path along which the social becomes the individual.*

For Vygotsky, SSD was a relational construct in which the current characteristics of a child interplayed with the interactions within his or her social structure to create a starting point for a new cycle of developmental changes. The SSD

1. Represents the initial background for major changes that happens in development during a given period of the child's life;
2. Forms a path along which an individual integrates social influence, thus determining new psychological characteristics of the child;
3. Is capable of powerfully facilitating or substantially disturbing the child's development by defining the child's way of life, social connections, and the peculiarities of consciousness; and
4. Is different in every social and historical situation: the activities through which the child's needs are being met are determined by the adults' cultural expectations regarding the child's gender, age, etc., and the adults' social/cultural means of impacting on a child.

Vygotsky made clear that the SSD has its objective and subjective aspects. Objective characteristics of SSD could be described both qualitatively and quantitatively: physical health, quality of nutrition, family functionality, living conditions, age-appropriate schooling, etc. The objective component is the child's place in the system of social relations, which are characterized by certain rights and responsibilities, demands imposed on personal behavior, and social expectations that have a historical nature and are developed by society in accordance with cultural ideas of child's psychological development.

The subjective aspect is the child's personal experience of the current situation that can be estimated and described as his or her attitudes, expectations, anxieties, self-perception, etc. The subjective component represents the child's "internal position"—the term used by Vygotsky and is close in many aspects to the "internal working model" proposed by Bowlby (1988). It is the system of internal factors that interprets and mediates social influences and defines the child's attitude toward his objective position in society. It is not enough to change the objective status of a child to accomplish the change in his psychological development; it requires a modified perception and interpretation of the new position by the child him or herself (Gindis & Kozulin, 2007; Lubovsky, 2009).

Further, Vygotsky maintained that the internal position of a child is realized through the perception of a leading activity (e.g., learning, socialization) that determines the psychological development within specific age stages. The SSD is defined by the child's connectedness with close adults (parents or other immediate caregivers), "social" adults (teachers, counselors), and peers (friends, classmates). The role of each agent of interaction changes at different developmental stages depending on the specificity of age-related circumstances.

These theoretical conceptualizations of Vygotsky have tremendous significance in the rehabilitation and remediation of international adoptees. The objective and subjective parameters of SSD can dramatically change any child's life as a result of man-made or natural disasters or changes in family life, such as divorce or untimely death. There may be favorable occurrences as well, such as an adoption into a loving and caring middle-class family. The lives of children adopted from overseas orphanages objectively change drastically and for the better, according to the prevailing "common sense." A subjective perception of such change is a different matter (Gindis, 1998).

Objectively, the SSD is radically different between orphanage and adoptive family, from inmates' group to family interaction, from one set of cultural arrangements to completely different ones, from one language to another, from the matter diet and physical conditions of living, the list can go on and on. A family has different expectations for the child's functioning, reacts differently to the child's behavior, etc. "Internal model" and survival patterns of behavior that were so deeply embedded into the child's psyche are challenged and tested by a new SSD. The changes in SSD occur literally overnight and are so radical that they may be subjectively traumatic by themselves.

Vygotsky suggested that with time, the parent's role, exceedingly important in the early childhood, gives way to interactions with peers that become particularly important in adolescence. Intra- and intergroup processes of communication with peers, rather than didactic interaction with parents, would determine the propagation of cultural experience and personality development under the influence of environmental contexts. Currently, the idea is widely accepted that both child-parent and child-peer communications determine the psychological development of a child (Bronfenbrenner, 2005).

Social Connectedness of a Child as a Major Factor of Development

Connectedness is a state of being socially related to a significant degree to a person or a group, and being accepted and integrated into this bond is meaningful for the child's relationship (Baumeister & Leary, 1995). The idea of pivotal significance of social connectedness for normal development is not something new or extraordinary in neuroscience: social connectedness as a crucial part of human development is accentuated in practically all modern theoretical developmental systems, such as Vygotsky's social-cultural theory (1987, 1993, 1998), Bowlby's attachment theory (1988), Bandura's social-learning theory (1977), Bronfenbrenner's ecological model (1998), and Bruner's learning theory (1996), just to list a few. As Cozolino coined (2014, p. xvii), "*The brain is a social organ of adaptation built through interactions with others.*"

Social connectedness with the mother has a special significance and is the prerequisite to appropriate social/emotional development and mental health of the child. In her well-known studies, M. Ainsworth described roughly three ways in which infants shape their behavior in regards to their caregivers: secure, anxious/avoidant, and ambivalent (Ainsworth, 1964, 1989) She explained that all these patterns are the product of different caregivers' responsiveness to the child. Secure infants tend to grow up able to rely on their emotions and thoughts to help them determine their reactions to any given situation. If children are exposed to unmanageable stress and their caregivers do not actively help modulate their arousal (due to being absent, impaired, neglectful, etc.) as frequently happens in dysfunctional families and orphanages, the children are unable to organize and categorize their experiences in a coherent fashion. These children are likely to become intolerably distressed, without the sense that an external environment can and should provide relief. Not being able to rely on their caregivers, these children experience excessive anxiety, fear, and anger, often resulting in aggressive or dissociative states. These frightened and hyper-aroused children can neither regulate their emotional states themselves nor compensate for their lack of affect regulation by relying on others to help them. The early patterns produced by a lack of social support and attachment have powerful effects throughout a child's life because they tend to establish a prototype of how people process subsequent stressful information (Baumeister & Leary, 1995).

As described by Cozolino (2014, pp. 116–117),

> early bonding and attachment experiences result in a cascade of biochemical processes that stimulate and enhance the growth and connectivity of neural networks throughout the brain. On the other hand, withdrawal from those on whom the baby depends for biological stimulation and growth causes distress, pain, and anxiety. Face-to-face interactions activate the child's sympathetic nervous system and increase oxygen consumption, energy metabolism, and gene expression. Healthy attachment requires from a caregiver appropriate reciprocal social exchange, positive emotional involvement, sensitivity, and affinity.

The transposition of maternal behavior into the biological structure of the brain presents a mechanism underlying the correlations between caregiving and subsequent physical and mental health. It gradually comes to the forefront of our understanding that the deficiency in social connectedness, regardless of the used "tags" (from attachment to social/emotional interactions, to individualized interpersonal relationships, etc.), is the major cause of many observed delays, disorders, and malfunctioning in human beings.

As was discussed in the previous chapter, a lack of or a distorted social connectedness is the major trauma-producing factor in IAPI children. Being exposed to unpredictable violence, repeated abandonment, and institutional care with its "structural neglect," IAPI children learn to cope with threatening events and emotions by maladaptive means (e.g., restricting their processing of what is happening around them). As a result, when they confront challenging situations, they may not be able to produce a coherent, proper response. These children have great difficulty regulating their emotions, managing stress, developing concern for others, and using language to solve problems. In order to cope, some IAPI children attempt to exert some control, often by disconnecting from social relationships or by acting coercively toward others. Studies have documented that maltreated children are either hypersensitive or avoidant in response to negative emotional stimuli and are likely to interpret positive emotions as ambiguous (D'Andrea, Ford, Stolbach, Spinazzola, & van der Kolk, 2012).

Psychological Tools and Mediated Learning

The concept of "psychological tools" is one of the cornerstones of Vygotsky's sociocultural theory of development. Just as humans invent mechanical tools to extend their physical capabilities, Vygotsky proposed that humankind also invents cultural or *psychological tools* to extend our powers of mind. Psychological tools are the symbolic cultural artifacts— signs, symbols, alphabets, written texts, maps, formulas, diagrams, etc., and most fundamentally, language—that enable human beings to master psychological functions, such as memory, perception, and attention, etc., in ways appropriate to our cultures. These cultural artifacts aim not only at mastering and transforming the external world but also at converting our natural psychological capacities into high-order psychological functions, such as abstract reasoning, voluntary attention, complex memorization, self-regulated goal-oriented behavior, and cooperation or competition with others. (Vygotsky, 1987, 1993). Vygotsky argued that higher psychological functions emerge from social communication as society transforms "natural" psychological functions into "cultural" ones. Adults teach these tools to children during day-to-day activities, and the children internalize them, so later the psychological tools can help students advance their own development.

Mediated learning is the special interaction between a child and an adult, who may be a parent, teacher, coach, counselor, or event older sibling. The concept of mediated learning was introduced by Vygotsky and later elaborated by R. Feuerstein (1997, 2003) and his associates. The mediating agent selects, enhances, focuses, and otherwise organizes stimuli for the child in order to improve the child's functioning and abilities. Through this process, the learners acquire behavior patterns, awareness, and strategies that in turn enhance their capacity to advance further. Mediation occurs through human interaction, and this shared learning/teaching activity enables learners to incorporate a great variety of orientations and strategies into their behavioral repertoire. In turn, new strategies for learning constitute a prerequisite for higher-order mental operations. Mediation is a key tool for transferring human knowledge and values from one generation to the other: interruption and/or lacking of this process result in failure to develop high psychological functions in a child.

Vygotsky stated that with a lack of mediation in mastering the psychological tools, individuals with normally developed natural abilities, such as spontaneous attention, simple memorization, practical problem solving, or imitative behavior, may nevertheless remain deprived of the important means of development offered by their culture. These subjects, in his terminology, exhibit cultural "primitivity," displaying behaviors similar to those with organic-based limitations. Vygotsky gave the following example. A child was asked, "How do a tree and a log differ?"

The child answered, "I have not seen a tree. I swear I haven't seen one." When shown a linden tree that stands under the window, he answered, "This is a linden" (Vygotsky, 1993, p. 46). Vygotsky commented that from the point of view of primitive logic, the child was right, no one had ever seen "a tree," all we had seen were lindens, chestnuts, ashes, and so on. "A tree" is a product of cultural development, when a word becomes not only a substitute for a concrete object, but it represents a class of objects, being cognitive generalization.

Cultural "primitivity" may coexist with neurological, cognitive, or physical impairments. However, while the acquisition of cultural tools can compensate for underdeveloped or impaired natural functions, even the normal development of natural functions cannot guarantee the establishment of higher mental abilities without mediated learning and the employment of cultural tools (Kozulin & Presseisen, 1995).

In the pre-adoption histories of IAPI children, we see the extreme case of a lack of mediated learning and a deprivation of basic psychological tools. Being born in dysfunctional, poverty stricken, and often abusive families and living in institutions where "systemic neglect" is the major attribute, IAPI children, particularly those adopted after the age of 5, present as an unfortunate "natural experiment," confirming Vygotsky's theoretical conjecture about psychological tools and mediated learning. Using Vygotsky's paradigm, we can state that IAPI children, due to severe neglect and deprivation during their formative years, have been deprived of both the "psychological tools" and "mediated learning," essential for the development of higher psychological functions. The already traumatized children in institutions have been culturally deprived of mastering psychological tools for their own mental processes: they have been delayed in the development of their high-order thinking, volition, and self-regulation of emotions and behavior (Gindis, 2003).

Cultural Difference and Cultural Deprivation

For international adoptees, especially for children adopted after their fifth birthday, the issue of *cultural difference vs. cultural deprivation* has crucial significance because both the cause of trauma and the means of rehabilitation are predominantly sociocultural in nature.

Numerous cross-cultural studies have been focused on so-called normative (typical) behavior and cognition, while the functioning of children with special needs was interpreted on an individual level without the involvement of cultural categories. A breakthrough came in the works of the Israeli psychologist R. Feuerstein and his associates (1997, 2003). They placed the concept of cultural difference and cultural deprivation at the very center of their theory of performance for children with special needs. As observed by A. Kozulin (2003), both Vygotsky and Feuerstein faced similar practical tasks: Vygotsky was challenged to create a special education system in post-revolutionary Russia under the conditions of sociocultural dislocation and the educational deprivation of large masses of children. Feuerstein was entrusted with finding educational solutions in the 1950s and 1960s for thousands of new immigrant children in Israel who were also, for the most part, educationally deprived and dislocated from their familiar sociocultural milieu. In the US and Western Europe, similar problems became recognized much later with the influx of internationally adopted post-institutionalized children in the late 1990s and first decade of the 21st century.

Let us consider a hypothetical, but close to reality, situation that I have observed in my clinical practice many times. Two 7-year-old boys began second grade in suburban Philadelphia. Both arrived from Poland; one was an immigrant child while the other was adopted from a Poland orphanage. The parents of the first child (both university-educated professionals but with limited English) explain to the school authorities that the boy has just finished the first grade in Poland and is anxious to begin learning in the new country. The adoptive mother of the second boy, a teacher herself, describes the situation with her new son, who had never been in school, because in his native land, the orphanage counselors didn't think the boy was ready for a formal education.

A year later, the immigrant boy is perfectly fluent in conversational English, does well in academic subjects, and even serves as his grandmother's translator when needed. Accepted by his classmates, in his teacher's opinion, he is pretty well adjusted socially, although not without some difficulties, expected for a newcomer.

The second boy is considered for special education. His conversational English is functional, but he has significant difficulties with mastering even the fundamentals of literacy in English. He has failed most of his subjects and seems unmotivated to learn. Socially, he presents certain behavior issues, alternating between withdrawal and aggression.

According to Vygotsky-Feuerstein's model, the first child's difficulties originate in the differences between the American and Polish culture and education. His cognitive and academic skills, however, allow him to overcome the initial hurdles and adapt to the new culture. For the second boy, the problems lay not only in the differences between educational systems but also in a lack of "psychological tools": there is not much he can transfer into his new educational environment because of his initial cultural background of deprivation. Like the majority of post-orphanage international adoptees, he belongs to the culturally deprived group. In other words, the success of the first child can be attributed to the sufficient experience with mediated learning he received from his family and his native country's educational system, while the difficulties of the second child were rooted in the absence of adequate mediated learning in his institutional background when he was forced to rely almost exclusively on his natural abilities.

Kozulin (Gindis & Kozulin, 2007) suggested that these two aspects, "psychological tools" and "mediated learning," should be integrated into one matrix. The following diagram in Table 3.1, developed by A. Kozulin (Gindis & Kozulin, 2007), presents a schematic view of possible relationships between problems in natural and cultural development:

Table 3.1 Psychological Tools and Mediated Learning

A. Mediated learning is adequate. Higher-level symbolic tools are available and internalized as psychological tools.	B. Mediated learning is adequate. Higher-level symbolic tools are unavailable.
C. Higher-level symbolic tools are available but fail to be internalized as psychological tools. Mediated learning is adequate in activities that do not require higher-level symbolic tools.	D. Mediated learning is insufficient. Higher-level symbolic tools are unavailable.

In my clinical work with children from immigrant families and IAPI children, I have observed that most children from immigrant families moving to the US and Canada fit into section A of the matrix and, to a lesser degree, into sections B and C. The majority of IAPI children match section D, and the minority, to a certain degree, fit into sections C and D.

Concept of "Zone of Proximal Development" and IAPI Children

Many years well before Vygotsky, thousands of teachers and parents intuitively felt and actually observed that with the proper assistance from an adult or a more advanced peer, a child is capable of much more learning than on his or her own. Vygotsky elevated this observation to a theoretical generalization known as the "Zone of Proximal Development" (ZPD). He stated that the process of properly guided assistance brings about abilities that have been in the process of emerging (developing) and have not yet matured and revealed itself. He defined the "Zone of Proximal Development" (Vygotsky, 1978, p. 86) as *"the distance between the actual developmental level as determined by independent problem solving and the level of potential development as determined through problem-solving under adult guidance, or in collaboration with more capable peers."*

The ZPD is one of Vygotsky's ideas that has a direct bearing on practice, both in psychological testing and in school instruction. The ZPD is often depicted as a three-layered dynamic environment (Table 3.2):

Table 3.2 Zone of Proximal Development Chart

The first layer encompasses knowledge and skills that are either well known to a learner or those he can master on his own.

The second layer represents what is not known or mastered yet, but a learner has the potential to acquire new knowledge and master new skills under the guidance of a knowledgeable and sympathetic instructor, formal and informal. This position represents the environment that is the most productive for learning and development—this is the "Zone of Proximal Development."

The third layer is an area of knowledge and skills that at the moment cannot be learned and mastered by a learner, even with the most skillful assistance, and are in a person's zone of frustration and discomfort.

Vygotsky's idea of the ZPD reflects on the psychological mechanism of transition from the social (shared) forms of mental processes to their individual forms. Vygotsky believed in the inseparable unity of the intellectual and the emotional, and his proposal of ZPD includes a positive emotional background and encouragement for a learner. In terms of individual differences, the depth of a ZPD varies, reflecting a child's cognitive learning potential, motivation, and emotional stability as determined by the interplay of biological and social factors in the child's background.

It is important to note that Vygotsky actually did not elaborate the issue of instructional methodology for creating ZPD; it was done by other psychologists and educators. Thus, the concept of "scaffolding" (guided assistance) was introduced by Wood, Bruner, and Ross (1976, p. 90), who define scaffolding as a process "that enables a child or novice to solve a task or achieve a goal that would be beyond his unassisted efforts."

As the authors note, scaffolds require the adults "controlling those elements of the task that are initially beyond the learner's capability, thus permitting him to concentrate upon and complete only those elements that are within his range of competence" (p. 90).

Actually, there is no "universal" or "the best on the market" methodology for implementing the ZPD concept. The principal method is to continually adjust the level of scaffolding in response to the learner's level of performance utilizing different specific methods, such as modeling a skill, providing hints or cues, adapting material or activity, and running "dynamic" assessment within the joint/shared activities with a child (Gindis & Karpov, 2000; Gindis & Lidz, 2003). The discussion of specific methodologies of operating within the ZPD is beyond the scope of this chapter.

In order to use ZPD and scaffolding techniques successfully, it's critical to know a particular IAPI child's current level of knowledge and skills. Without this information, the teacher or parent won't be able to discover the ZPD or provide effective scaffolding support. That is why initial screening in the native language is so important for IAPI children.

I found that each IAPI school-aged child has a different ZPD for each academic subject. Thus, orphans from Russia typically are more advanced in math due to Russia's effective math teaching methodology (Karp & Vogeli, 2011). I will never forget an angry letter I once received from an elementary schoolteacher in upstate New York. She received my report of a newly adopted child from Russia who had fetal alcohol syndrome, was recognized in his native country as a child with intellectual disability, and had a composite score below 70 on the nonverbal test (UNIT). While working with this 8-year-old boy, I came to the conclusion that he indeed met all major characteristics of a person qualified for the intellectual disability classification. I had completed his educational testing according to the Russian curriculum and given him the math tests WJ-lll Achievement battery with calculation, math fact fluency, math reasoning, and math word problems translated into Russian, as the child had been in the country for only three weeks. I found that although he barely made the end of the first grade in math according to the Russian curriculum, he performed at the beginning of the fourth grade in math according to US educational tests. That is what made the teacher upset: "How can you call this student intellectually disable when his math is better than any of my second graders?" she asked. I had to explain to her that school-age adoptees from Russia and China routinely have high math scores, because children with cognitive limitations still can be taught math at a surprising level to American teachers.

The ZPD in the IAPI children is qualitatively different from the same in their "typical" classmates. Thus, while in the activities of daily living, many IAPI children can be above age expectations, in cognitive/academic language mastering, general academic learning (with possible exceptions in certain subjects), and social skills, their ZPD is rather narrow (please see a more detailed discussion in Chapter 7).

One of the most typical obstacles in using the ZPD methodology with IAPI children is their "learned helplessness." In its origin, it is a survival skill, part of a post-orphanage behavior syndrome: a child in an institution quickly learns that he should present as helpless in order to attract more attention from an adult. Some, if not the majority, of post-institutionalized children have deeply internalized this position and are able to appeal to teachers and parents with demonstrated helplessness. Many of these children actually have the needed skills or knowledge, but may be resistant to any attempt to encourage them to reveal knowledge or skill and act independently. Sometimes the line between learned helplessness and real need may be rather thin. But learning in ZPD is not possible without properly accepting help from an instructor or more advanced peer. As a result of demonstrated learned helplessness, such IAPI children may receive too much help, which causes the student to be a passive, uninvolved, and uninterested learner. Because of their emotional fragility, IAPI children are more vulnerable to the mismatch between their academic readiness and level of instruction; they are less robust in their ability to withstand the stress related to school performance, and they are less self-sufficient in overcoming the emotional strain, which is a part of competing in the school environment. Indeed, educational professionals who need to determine IAPI children's ZPD have to walk a fine line, providing them with intense and focused remediation, and at the same time not overwhelming them with unreasonable expectations and demands.

Deviations in Physical Growth and Physiological Maturation in IAPI Children

The children reared in orphanages tend to be smaller in height, weight, and head and chest circumference (Miller, 2005; Johnson & Gunnar, 2011). The "psychosocial short stature" hypothesis (Johnson & Gunnar, 2011) states that children exposed to social-emotional neglect display growth deficiencies called "psychosocial dwarfism," also known as "psychogenic stress dwarfism" (Bowden & Hopwood, 2008). As stated by Gunnar (2001), the growth deficiency is likely to result from the hyperactivity caused by the corticotrophin released by the hormone-hypothalamus-pituitary-adrenal axis, which reduces the growth both centrally and peripherally. The social and emotional deprivation, neglect, and abuse coexist with deficiencies in nutrition, physical exercise, medical care, and other factors that delay growth. The disorder progresses while the person stays in a stress-producing environment, but regular growth may resume when the source of stress is removed. This disorder is rather rare in the population at large; it was considered exotic (Hall & Adelson, 2005) until the beginning of massive international adoption from Eastern European countries, particularly from Romania. It was found that as a group, IAPI children average more than one standard deviation below the level expected of noninstitutionalized children with respect to their physical growth (Van IJzendoorn, Bakermans-Kranenburg, & Juffer, 2007; Sonuga-Barke, Edmund, & Kreppner, 2012). This deviation was found even in children from institutions that reportedly provided adequate general nutrition and medical care (The St. Petersburg-USA Orphanage Research Team, 2008). After adoption, these children, on average, have shown substantial catchup in growth (Van IJzendoorn, et al., 2007). Further, growth can be improved if the psychosocial environment of the orphanage is improved without changing nutrition (The St. Petersburg-USA Orphanage Research Team, 2008; Sonuga-Barke et al., 2012).

In their comprehensive review of the phenomenon, Johnson and Gunnar (2011) explain that the nutritional deficiencies contribute to the suppression of the growth hormone, but psychosocial growth failure within institutional settings is mostly attributed to social deprivation and neglect (trauma). The authors observed that, while a catchup in height and weight is rapid after adoption, many factors, particularly early progression through puberty, compromise the progress. A high incidence of growth failure in institutionalized children is a universal finding with every cohort reported to date showing at least moderate suppression of height, weight, and head circumference (Van IJzendoorn & Juffer, 2006).

Another physiological consequence of psychosocial deprivation during their growth period in IAPI girls (and to a lesser extent in boys) is a much higher rate of early puberty, even when compared to children of the same ethnicity (Teilmann et al., 2009). Precocious puberty is sexual maturation in boys and girls that occurs at an unusually early age, at least 2.5 standard deviations below the mean age at onset of puberty in their peers. One large study in Denmark (Teilmann et al., 2009) reported that internationally adopted girls run a significantly increased risk of developing precocious puberty. Initially, the most popular explanation was that children adopted from developing countries may arrive at their new homes in a chronically undernourished state, but in the following months, the improved nutritional conditions determine a catchup in linear and weight growth that may trigger the onset of puberty. However, there are several research publications that link precocious puberty to early childhood adversity: not only a change of diet but also a combination of age at adoption, genetic factors, nutritional status prior to adoption, and pre- and post-adoption growth patterns (Bergevin, Bukowski, & Karavasilis, 2003; Romans, Martin, Gendall, & Herbison, 2003; Mendle, Leve, Van Ryzin, Natsuaki, & Ge, 2011, 2014). In the population at large in Western cultures, early puberty is related to higher rates of mental health problems, especially depression, and earlier sexual activity (Sonuga-Barke et al., 2012). Precocious puberty in IAPI children was connected to psychosocial maladjustment, increased risk-taking behavior, and low final height following early pubertal development.

Sensitive Periods in Development and a Complex Childhood Trauma

It is a well-established scientific fact that in human development, there are periods of time during which certain experiences are necessary to fully develop an individual's physical, mental, language, and social capacities. Development during these periods sets the stage for everything that follows: less than optimal use of these periods will result in delays and distortions in the evolution of particular abilities, and the absence or presence of specific social experiences can have a permanent effect on the physiological functioning of the brain. Moreover, if the influences do not occur, the individuals may lose some of their native potential capacity for a specific psychological function. These periods are called "critical," "sensitive," or in the context of adversity, "vulnerable" (Greenough, Black, & Wallace, 1987). The researchers still wildly disagree on the role of specific timing, duration, and limitations of sensitive periods in the different aspects of development (Bailey, Bruer, Symons, & Lichtman, 2001).

In the context of this book, the issue of the effect of the social environment on plasticity in the earliest attachment relationships is particular important. All infants have the capacity, indeed the genetic predisposition, to form strong attachments to their primary caregivers (McCrory et al., 2010; Hertzman, 2012). But if the child's caregivers are unresponsive or the attachment process is disrupted, the child's ability to form any healthy relationships during his life may be impaired. Social deprivation in early life can cause vulnerability to disorders of emotion regulation, cognitive function, and mental health (Pollak et al., 2010). As stated in a number of research publications, exposure to severe neglect and deprivation during the first two years of life is potentially sufficient to produce the higher rates of long-term behavioral, emotional, and cognitive problems (Van der Kolk, 2003; Van der Vegt, Van der Ende, Ferdinand, Verhulst, & Tiemeier, 2009; Shonkoff & Garner, 2012). Further, the literature on the adoption of previously institutionalized children shows that institutionalization that ends by 6 months, or in some cases 12 months, does not have as deleterious longer-term effects as institutionalization until the second birthday does (Gunnar, 2001; MacLean, 2003; Rutter et al., 2009).

Besides the age at which a traumatic negative impact occurs, the consequences go hand in hand with the severity of the pre-adoption experience. Thus, children adopted from arguably the worst Romanian orphanages in the 1990s at around 6 months had shown significant multiple long-term problems (Kreppner et al., 2007; Stevens, van Rooij, & Jovanovic, 2016). Children from Russian orphanages adopted around 18 months old showed extreme behaviors and immature social skills (Hawk & McCall, 2011; Merz & McCall, 2010). For children adopted from China, the critical period was around the second birthday (Gunnar, 2001). The bottom line is that the age of exposure and the severity of traumatic influences increase the risk of impairments with learning, memory, and the ability to regulate emotions and behavior. These effects may well be observed after as little as 6 months in severely depriving orphanages and within the first two years for many other institutions.

However, the statement "the earlier adoption—the better outcome" enthusiastically proclaimed by some researches (see Bakermans-Kranenburg, Van IJzendoorn, & Juffer, 2008; Almas, 2012 ; Compton, 2016) is not as unquestionably accurate as it appears at first glance. How can one explain that there is a significant number of IAPI children who spent not only infant and toddler years in orphanages but also most of their preschool and even school years there—the so-called older adoptees—who still show amazing recovery and near normal functioning? On the other hand, the number of those adopted before their second birthday that still had significant delays and disorders is high too (Juffer & Van IJzendoorn, 2005; Juffer, Palacios, Lemare, van IJzendoorn, & Verhulst, 2011). There is an obvious need to identify a connection between trauma, various sensitive periods, and specific psychological functions to find that mysterious "point of no return" when the consequences of trauma have emerged and stabilized. There is still no definite answer to whether there is a sensitive period during which the exposure to "toxic stress" produces the maximum developmental damage in international adoptees.

The issue of "sensitive" or, in the framework of trauma, "vulnerable" periods of early childhood will be discussed in this book in all chapters that follow in relation to cognition, language, and learning in IAPI children. Similar to attachment and, broader, social/emotional functioning, other psychological functions and capabilities have sensitive periods of development mercilessly damaged by neglect, deprivation, and abandonment. Thus, lack of mediated learning in the first years of life in IAPI children leads to cumulative cognitive deficit (Chapter 4) and deficiency in verbal input from the birth to preschool years produces language delays and disorders (Chapter 5), as well as academic failure, particularly beyond the elementary school in so many IAPI children (Chapter 7).

Developmental "Catchup" and Long-Lasting Deficiencies in IAPI Children

In the developmental context, "catching up" and "long-lasting deficiencies" present one of the most controversial notions in the field of psychology of international adoption. On one hand, many, if not the majority, of research papers on this subject are excited about the amazing abilities of IAPI children to improve their functioning to reach the age-appropriate standards (see a comprehensive review in van IJzendoorn & Juffer, 2006; Compton, 2016).

On the other hand, there are a significant number of quality publications proving that the "catchup" is only relative in regard to the initial status of IAPI children (Hildyard & Wolfe, 2002; Gindis, 2005; van der Vegt et al., 2009; Welsh & Viana, 2012). As presented in a number of publications, after spending years with an adoptive family, IAPI children on average score below expectations on general mental tests and exhibit a variety of deficiencies in executive functioning: problems with attention, self-regulation, working memory, and planning. They continue to have attachment, relationship, and social engagement difficulties, as well as a variety of internalized and externalized behavior problems, especially during adolescence. It is particularly applicable to the so-called older adoptees, those exposed to traumatic experiences for a longer period of time: they display higher rates of deficiencies and problems in several domains (Juffer & Van IJzendoorn, 2005; Tieman, Van der Ende, & Verhulst, 2005; van Londen, Juffer, & van IJzendoorn, 2007; Rutter et al., 2009; Juffer et al., 2011; Pollak et al., 2010; Hawk & McCall, 2011).

It is possible to summarize the major findings made within the last 30 years in relation to the developmental outcomes in international adoptees:

- Initially, the children demonstrated significant delays in many domains of their development.
- The majority showed developmental improvement following adoption.
- The catchup in many cases was inconsistent and incomplete.
- An evident minority (no statistic exists) demonstrated persistent, permanent deficits in one or more developmental domains.

I am not aware of any specific meta-analysis on what facilitates or inhibits developmental recovery in IAPI children, but my own account on this matter, based on about 30 years of clinical experience, includes the following:

1. The degree of initial impairment: cognitive limitations, psychiatric disorders, medical problems, and other special needs.
2. Birth country and the related pre-adoptive experiences: indeed, donor countries vary considerably in terms of quality of institutional care, and children from low-quality orphanages show greater developmental deficits. According to a number of research reports, children adopted from India and Eastern Europe, particularly from Romania and, to a somewhat lesser degree, from Russia, had more pre-adoptive adversity than children adopted from South Korea and China. Central American countries have a significant diversity in pre-adoption care as well (Pomerleau et al., 2005; van Londen et al., 2007; Odenstad et al., 2008; Van den Dries, Juffer, van IJzendoorn, & Bakermans-Kraneburg, 2009; Welsh & Viana, 2012).
3. The age at adoption and so-called dose-response factor: the higher the dose of trauma, the more potentially damaging the effects. This point of view was expressed in many research publications (see Judge, 2003; Bakermans-Kranenburg et al., 2008; Rutter et al., 2009; Welsh & Viana, 2012). However, findings related to the age and duration of institutional experience as a factor in developmental trajectories of children after adoption are inconsistent. I would agree with Welch & Viana that "it is possible that other factors, such as the quality of care the child received prior to adoption, or biological risks factors, such as premature birth or prenatal substance exposure, are more powerful predictors of outcome than age at placement" (p. 261).

4. The quality and quantity of post-adoption remediation and rehabilitation, the strength of social connectedness with the adoptive family, and the post-adoption social/cultural environment as the decisive forces.
5. It is likely that developmental catchup is domain specific: the existing data suggest that there are certain domains of overall functioning affected more profoundly and persistently than others: specifically, cognitive competency and social/emotional self-regulation recover more slowly and, in some cases, may never be rehabilitated up to the age expectations (Almas, 2012; Beckett et al., 2006).

In sum, the research publications and clinical practice are united in that the delayed development and observed deviations from the expected developmental level of functioning in IAPI children are a synergetic effect of a host of traumatic factors that negatively affect the post-adoption developmental outcomes. At the same time, IAPI children's development is positively influenced by post-adoptive remediation and rehabilitation, adoptive family nurturing, and social/cultural enrichment. It appears that the age of adoption, quality of adoptive family social support, and constructive social connectedness outside of the family are the most valid predictors of the positive dynamic of IAPI children's development after their adoptions.

References

Ainsworth, M. (1964). Patterns of attachment behavior shown by the infant in interaction with his mother. *Merrill-Palmer Quarterly of Behavior and Development, 10*(1), 51–58.

Ainsworth, M. (1989). Attachments beyond infancy. *American Psychologist, 44*(4), 709–716.

Almas, A. (2012). Effects of early intervention and the moderating effects of brain activity on institutionalized children's social skills at age 8. *Proceedings of the National Academy of Sciences, 109*, 17228–17231.

Bailey, B., Bruer, J. T., Symons, F. J., & Lichtman, J. W. (Eds.) (2001). *Critical thinking about critical periods.* Baltimore: Paul H. Brookers Publishing.

Bakermans-Kranenburg, M., Van IJzendoorn, M., & Juffer, F. (2008). Earlier is better: A meta-analysis of 70 years of intervention improving cognitive development in institutionalized children. *Monographs of the Society for Research of Child Development, 73*, 279–293.

Bandura, A. (1977). *Social learning theory.* Englewood Cliffs, NJ: Prentice-Hall.

Baumeister, R. F., & Leary, M. R. (1995). The need to belong: Desire for interpersonal attachments as a fundamental human motivation. *Psychological Bulletin, 117*, 497–529.

Beckett, C., Maughan, B., Rutter, M., Castle, J., Colvert, E., Groothues, C., & Sonuga-Barke, E. J. S. (2006). Do the effects of early deprivation on cognition persist into early adolescence? Findings from the English and Romanian adoptee study. *Child Development, 77*, 696–711.

Bergevin, T., Bukowski, W., & Karavasilis, L. (2003). Child sexual abuse and pubertal timing: Implications for long-term psychosocial adjustment. In C. Hayward (Ed.), *Gender differences at puberty* (pp. 187–216). Cambridge: Cambridge University Press.

Bowden, M. L., & Hopwood, N. J. (2008). Psychosocial dwarfism: Identification, intervention, and planning. *Social Work in Health Care, 7*(3), 15–36.

Bowlby, J. (1988). *A secure base: Parent-child attachment and healthy human development.* New York: Basic Books.

Bronfenbrenner, U. (2005). *Making human beings human: Bioecological perspectives on human development.* Thousand Oaks, CA: Sage.

Bronfenbrenner, U. (1998). The ecology of developmental processes. In W. Damon & R. M. Lerner (Eds.), *Handbook of child psychology: Theoretical models of human development* (5th ed., Vol. 1, pp. 993–1028). New York: Wiley & Sons.

Bruner, J. S. (1996). *The culture of education.* Cambridge, MA: Harvard University Press.

Champagne, D. L., Bagot, R. C., Hasselt, F., van Ramakers, G., Meaney, M. J., de Kloet, E. R., & Krugers, H. (2008). Maternal care and hippocampal plasticity: Evidence for experience-dependent structural plasticity, altered synaptic functioning, and differential responsiveness to glucocorticoids and stress. *The Journal of Neuroscience, 28,* 6037–6045.

Cozolino, L. (2014). *The neuroscience of human relationships: Attachment and the developing social brain* (2nd ed.). New York: W.W. Norton and Co.

D'Andrea, W., Ford, J., Stolbach, B., Spinazzola, J., & van der Kolk, B. A. (2012). Understanding interpersonal trauma in children: Why we need a developmentally appropriate trauma diagnosis. *American Orthopsychiatric Association, 82*(2), 187–200.

Feuerstein, R., & Gross, S. (1997). The learning potential assessment device. In D. Flanagan, et al. (Eds.), *Contemporary intellectual assessment: Theories, tests, and issues.* New York: The Guilford Press.

Feuerstein, R., Rand, Y., Falik, L., & Feuerstein, R. (2003). *Dynamic assessment of cognitive modifiability.* Jerusalem: ICELP Press.

Fox, S. E., Levitt, P., & Nelson, C. A. (2010). How the timing and quality of early experiences influence the development of brain architecture. *Child Development, 81*(1), 28–40.

Gindis, B. (1998). Navigating uncharted waters: School psychologists working with internationally adopted post-institutionalized children. *Communiqué (National Association of School Psychologists),* September (Part I), 27(1), 6–9 and October (Part II), 27(2), 20–23.

Gindis, B. (2003). Remediation through education: Socio/cultural theory and children with special needs. Chapter 10 in A. Kozulin, B. Gindis, V. Ageyev, & S. Miller (Eds.), *Vygotsky's educational theory in cultural context* (pp. 200–222). New York: Cambridge University Press.

Gindis, B. (2005). Cognitive, language, and educational issues of children adopted from overseas orphanages. *Journal of Cognitive Education and Psychology, 4*(3), 290–315.

Gindis, B., & Karpov, Y. (2000). Dynamic assessment of the level of internalization of elementary school children's problem-solving activity. In C. S. Lidz & J. G. Elliott (Eds.), *Dynamic assessment: Prevailing models and applications* (pp. 133–154). Amsterdam: Elsevier Science.

Gindis, B., & Kozulin, A. (2007). Sociocultural theory and education of children with special needs: From defectology to remedial pedagogy. In H. Daniels, M. Cole, & J. Wertsch (Eds.), *The Cambridge companion to Vygotsky* (pp. 332–363). New York: Cambridge University Press.

Gindis, B., & Lidz, C. (2003). Dynamic assessment of the evolving cognitive functions in children. Chapter 5 in *Vygotsky's educational theory in cultural context* (pp. 99–116). New York: Cambridge University Press.

Greenough, W. T., Black, J. E., & Wallace, C. S. (1987). Experience and brain development. *Child Development, 58,* 539–559.

Gunnar, M. R. (2001). Effects of early deprivation: Findings from orphanage-reared infants and children. In C. A. Nelson & M. Luciana (Eds.), *Handbook of developmental cognitive neuroscience* (pp. 617–629). Cambridge, MA: The MIT Press.

Gunnar, M. R., & Quevedo, K. (2007). The neurobiology of stress and development. *Annual Review of Psychology, 58,* 145–173.

Hall, J., & Adelson, B. (2005). *Dwarfism: Medical and psychosocial aspects of profound short stature.* Baltimore: Johns Hopkins University Press.

Hawk, B. H., & McCall, R. B. (2011). Specific extreme behaviors of post-institutionalized Russian adoptees. *Developmental Psychology, 47*(3), 732–738.

Heim, C., & Binder, E. (2012). Current research trends in early life stress and depression: Review of human studies on sensitive periods, gene: Environment interactions, and epigenetics. *Experimental Neurology, 233*(1), 102–111.

Hertzman, C. (2012). Putting the concept of biological embedding in historical perspective. *Proceedings of the National Academy of Sciences, 109,* 17160–17167.

Hildyard, K. L., & Wolfe, D. A. (2002). Child neglect: Developmental issues and outcomes. *Child Abuse and Neglect, 26,* 679–695.

Johnson, D. E., & Gunnar, M. R. (2011). IV: Growth failure in institutionalized children. *Monographs of the Society for Research in Child Development, 76*(4), 92–126.

Judge, S. (2003). Developmental recovery and deficit in children adopted from Eastern European orphanages. *Child Psychiatry and Human Development, 34,* 49–62.

Juffer, F., Palacios, J., Lemare, L., van IJzendoorn, M., & Verhulst, F. (2011). II: Development of adopted children with histories of early adversity. *Monographs of the Society for Research in Child Development, 76,* 31–61.

Juffer, F., & Van IJzendoorn, M. H. (2005). Behavior problems and mental health referrals of international adoptees: A meta-analysis. *JAMA-Journal of the American Medical Association, 293*(20), 2501–2515.

Karp, A., & Vogeli, B. (2011). *Russian mathematics education: Programs and practices.* New York: Columbia University Press.

Kozulin, A. (2003). Psychological tools and mediated learning. In A. Kozulin, B. Gindis, V. Ageyev, & S. Miller (Eds.), *Vygotsky's educational theory in cultural context* (pp. 15–38). New York: Cambridge University Press.

Kozulin, A., & Presseisen, B. (1995). Mediated learning experience and psychological tools: Vygotsky's and Feuerstein's perspectives in a study of students' learning. *Educational Psychologist, 30,* 67–75.

Kreppner, J. M., Rutter, M., Beckett, C., Castle, J., Colvert, E., Groothues, C., & Sonuga-Barke, E. J. S. (2007). Normality and impairment following profound early institutional deprivation: A longitudinal follow-up into early adolescence. *Developmental Psychology, 43*(4), 931–946.

Lohmann, C., & Kessels, H. (2014). The developmental stages of synaptic plasticity. *The Journal of Physiology, 592*(1), 13–31.

Lubovsky, D. (2009). The concept of internal position in the cultural-historical perspective on studying the personality of the schoolchild. *Journal of Russian and East European Psychology, 47*(4), 87–96.

MacLean, K. (2003). The impact of institutionalization on child development. *Development and Psychopathology, 15*, 853–884.

McCrory, E., De Brito, S. A., & Viding, E. (2010). Research review: The neurobiology and genetics of maltreatment and adversity. *Journal Child Psychology and Psychiatry, 51*, 1079–1095.

McEwen, B. S. (2012). Brain on stress: How the social environment gets under the skin. *Proceedings of the National Academy of Sciences, 109*, 17180–17185.

McEwan, B. S., & Gianaros, P. J. (2010). Central role of the brain in stress and adaptations: Links to socioeconomic status, health, and disease. *Annals of the New York Academy of Sciences, 1186*, 190–222.

Mendle, J., Leve, L. D., Van Ryzin, M., & Natsuaki, M. N. (2014). Linking childhood maltreatment with girls' internalizing symptoms: Early puberty as a tipping point. *Journal of Research on Adolescence: The Official Journal of the Society for Research on Adolescence, 24*(4), 689–702.

Mendle, J., Leve, L. D., Van Ryzin, M., Natsuaki, M. N., & Ge, X. (2011). Associations between early life stress, child maltreatment, and pubertal development in foster care girls. *Journal of Research on Adolescence, 21*, 871–880.

Merz, E. C., & McCall, R. B. (2010). Behavior problems in children adopted from socially/emotionally depriving institutions. *Journal of Abnormal Child Psychology, 38*, 459–470.

Miller, J. (2005). *The handbook of international adoption medicine: A guide for physicians, parents, and provides.* New York: Oxford University Press.

Nelson, J. N., Kendall, G. E., & Shields, L. (2014). Neurological and biological foundations of children's social and emotional development: An integrated literature review. *The Journal of School Nursing, 30*(4), 240–250.

Odenstad, A., Hjern, A., Lindblad, F., Rasmussen, F., Vinnerljung, B., & Dalen, M. (2008). Does age at adoption and geographic origin matter? A national cohort study of cognitive test performance in adult inter-country adoptees. *Psychological Medicine, 38*, 1803–181.

Perry, B. D., Pollard, R., Blakely, T., Baker, W., & Vigilante, D. (1995). Childhood trauma, the neurobiology of adaptation and "use-dependent" development of the brain: How "states" become "traits" *Infant Mental Health Journal, 16*(4), 271–291.

Pollak, S. D., Nelson, C. A., Schlaak, M. F., Roeber, B. J., Wewerka, S. S., Wiik, K. L., & Gunnar, M. R. (2010). Neurodevelopmental effects of early deprivation in post-institutionalized children. *Child Development, 81*(1), 224–236.

Pomerleau, A., Malcuit, G., Chicoine, J., Séquin, R., Belhumeur, C., & Germain, P. (2005). Health status, cognitive and motor development of young children adopted from China, East Asia, and Russia across the first 6 months after adoption. *International Journal of Behavioral Development, 29,* 445–457.

Romans, S. E., Martin, M., Gendall, K., & Herbison, G. P. (2003). Age of menarche: The role of some psychosocial factors. *Psychological Medicine, 33,* 933–939.

Rutter, M., Beckett, C., Castle, J., Colvert, E., Kreppner, J., Mehta, M., & Sonuga-Barke, E. (2009). Effects of profound early institutional deprivation: An overview of findings from a UK longitudinal study of Romanian adoptees. In G. Wrobel & E. Neil (Eds.), *International advances in adoption research for practice.* Cambridge, MA: Wiley-Blackwell.

Shonkoff, J. P., & Garner, A. S. (2012). The lifelong effects of early childhood adversity and toxic stress. *Pediatrics, 129,* 232–246.

Sonuga-Barke, S., Edmund, J., & Kreppner, J. (2012). The development and care of institutionally reared children. *Child Development Perspectives, 6*(2), 174–180.

Stevens, J. S., van Rooij, S. J. H., & Jovanovic, T. (2016). Developmental contributors to trauma response: The importance of sensitive periods, early environment, and sex differences. In *Current topics in behavioral neurosciences* (pp. 1–22). Berlin, Heidelberg: Springer.

The St. Petersburg-USA Orphanage Research Team (2008). The effects of early social-emotional and relationship experience on the development of young children. *Monographs of the Society for Research in Child Development, 72*(3), vii–295. Publisher: John Wiley & Sons.

Teilmann, G., Petersen, J. H., Gormsen, M., Damgaard, K., Skakkebaek, N. E., & Jensen, T. K. (2009). Early puberty in internationally adopted girls: Hormonal and clinical markers of puberty in 276 girls examined biannually over two years. *Hormone Research in Pediatrics, 74*(4), 236–246.

Tieman, W., Van der Ende, J., & Verhulst, F. C. (2005). Psychiatric disorders in young adult intercountry adoptees: An epidemiological study. *American Journal of Psychiatry, 162*(3), 592–598.

Van der Kolk, B. (2003). The neurobiology of childhood trauma and abuse. *Child Adolescent Psychiatric Clinic of North America, 12,* 293–317.

Van der Vegt, E. J. M., Van der Ende, J., Ferdinand, R. F., Verhulst, F. C., & Tiemeier, H. (2009). Early childhood adversities and trajectories of psychiatric problems in adoptees: Evidence for long lasting effects. *Journal of Abnormal Child Psychology, 37,* 239–249.

Van IJzendoorn, M. H., Bakermans-Kranenburg, M., & Juffer, F. (2007). Plasticity of growth in height, weight and head circumference: Meta-analytic evidence for massive catch-up after international adoption. *Journal of Developmental and Behavioral Pediatrics, 28*(4), 334–343.

Van IJzendoorn, M. H., & Juffer, F. (2006). Adoption as intervention: Meta-analytic evidence for massive catch-up and plasticity in physical, socio-emotional and cognitive development: The Emanuel Miller memorial lecture 2006. *Journal of Child Psychology and Psychiatry, 47,* 1128–1245.

Van Londen, W., Juffer, F., & van IJzendoorn, M. (2007). Attachment, cognitive, and motor development in adopted children: Short-term outcomes after international adoption. *Journal of Pediatric Psychology, 32*(10), 1249–1258.

Van den Dries, L., Juffer, F., van IJzendoorn, M., & Bakermans-Kraneburg, M. (2009). Fostering security? A meta-analysis of attachment in adopted children. *Children and Youth Services Review, 31*(3), 410–421.

Vygotsky, L. S. (1978). *Mind in society: The development of higher psychological processes.* Cambridge, MA: Harvard University Press.

Vygotsky, L. S. (1987). *The collected works of L. S. Vygotsky. Volume 1: Problems of general psychology* (N. Minick, Trans. and R. W. Rieber & A. S. Carton, Eds.). New York: Plenum Press.

Vygotsky, L. S. (1993). *The collected works of L. S. Vygotsky. Volume 2: The fundamentals of defectology (Abnormal psychology and learning disabilities)* (J. E. Knox & C. B. Stevens, Trans. and R. W. Rieber & A. S. Carton, Eds.). New York: Plenum Press.

Vygotsky, L. S. (1998). *The collected works of L. S. Vygotsky. Volume 5: Child psychology* (R. W. Rieber, Ed.). New York: Plenum Press.

Welsh, J., & Viana, A. (2012). Developmental outcomes of internationally adopted children. *Adoption Quarterly, 15*(4), 241–264.

Wood, D. J., Bruner, J. S., & Ross, G. (1976). The role of tutoring in problem solving. *Journal of Child Psychiatry and Psychology, 17*, 89–100.

4 "Language Lost—Language Found" Experience

Distinct Pattern of Language Development in Internationally Adopted Post-Institutionalized Children

Introduction

With all the ethnic, cultural, and individual differences among international adoptees, there is one factor that is common to all of them: the language of the adoptive family is not their native tongue. Learning a new language is an inevitable part of being adopted internationally. In many IAPI children, this is a rather distressing experience related to an abrupt loss of the native language and a relatively slow acquisition of another language in a situation of ongoing stress of adjustment to a new physical and social/cultural environment. At the same time, language is an effective means of addressing trauma—it has multifaced applications and must be considered in any therapeutic work and remedial programming for IAPI children.

Language as a psychological function is one of the most powerful human abilities. At the same time, it is one of the most fragile and vulnerable of all of an individual's attributes. It is deeply rooted in human biology, yet, as no other psychological capacity, it depends on social/cultural milieu for its very existence and development. Language is a psychological function that mediates many of the other psychological competencies, such as perception, memory, cognition, social interaction, and goal-directed behavior, just to list a few. From the psychological perspective, there are four major domains of direct language application: communication, behavior regulation, learning, and a main medium of thinking/cognitive operations.

Language as a psychological utility is known for its distinctive "schedule of development" within the overall process of human physical growth, physiological maturity, and social adaptiveness. Advances in contemporary neuroscience lead us to believe that sensitive periods for different aspects of language functioning occur from birth to pre-puberty (Mayberry, & Lock, 2003; Sakai, 2005). The rate of early learning—literally the first months and years of life—determines the child's level of functioning for many years to come: what has not been mastered within certain developmental stages may not be totally compensated later in life (White, Hutka, Williams, & Moreno, 2013).

Inevitably, questions are generated: are there universal norms of language development, applicable to all children in all countries, in all socio/economic groups, in both genders? It is a well-known fact that children do not reach the same milestone in their language development on exactly the same schedule. Their developmental rate can vary by several months or even a year, and there is no evidence that "late talkers" end up as less fluent than "early talkers." Nevertheless, there are certain flexible markers of language acquisition, applicable to all cultures: from ages 3 to 5, children are bound to use language as their primary means of communication. If a child at the age of 5 can produce only a few dozen words that only his mother can understand, and grunts, points, and gestures to get what he wants, we would consider the child as having language problems.

Language can be acquired in a spontaneous and natural fashion; it can be learned in a systematic and planned way or can be mastered as a combination of both. IAPI children master new language as a by-product of life and shared activities with native speakers. The IAPI children receive formal instruction in their new language at school, but teachers are only one source of language acquisition, while adoptive parents, peers, media, and culture at large are the most influential facilitators of language learning. When IAPI children enter an unknown cultural and linguistic environment, learning language for them is no less than a survival effort: they have to acquire communicative language skills for normal functioning, as the entire process of adjustment is mediated by language. New language acquisition is the most crucial skill to be learned by an IAPI child in their first year in an adoptive family.

In order to discuss the issue of language functioning in IAPI children, I have to introduce related terminology used in the fields of linguistic, education, and psychology: bilingualism, circumstantial language learning, sequential monolingualism, first-language attrition, social/communicative language vs. cognitive/academic language acquisition, and language as a behavior regulator.

Bilingualism or Sequential Monolingualism

Are IAPI children bilingual individuals? The answer is a resounding "no." A common understanding of bilingualism includes functional use of more than one language within a developmentally appropriate and socially expected range of language skills (Baker, 2001). In this respect, a vast majority of IAPI children are not bilingual, or they may be bilingual for only a short period of time soon after adoption. They are monolingual at arrival (e.g., a 4-year-old girl with Chinese as her only language) and after several months, they are monolingual again; this time English only. There are, of course, a few exceptions, like older adolescents within sibling groups, but even in such cases, the loss or substantial deterioration of their first language skills is only a matter of time. In analogy with sequential bilinguals, when the second language is learned after the first one, the IAPI children can be called "sequential monolinguals," because after a short period of transitional "bilingualism," they are returned to the status of monolinguals for all practical purposes (Gindis, 1998, 1999a, 2005; Nicoladis & Grabois, 2002; Pearson, 2010; Scott, Roberts, & Glennen, 2011). The overwhelming majority of IAPI children use only English after a year in their adoptive families. Nevertheless, there is a tendency, particularly in school settings, to consider internationally adopted children as bilingual and to apply to them the insights, knowledge, and practices that have been accumulated regarding language acquisition in bilingual persons (Meese, 2002). Viewing these children as bilingual is one of the most damaging misconceptions in our educational and mental health systems.

"Circumstantial" English Language Learners

IAPI children are the extreme case of a so-called circumstantial model of language learning. "Circumstantial" learners of another language are individuals who, because of their circumstances, find that they must learn another language in order to function in a society they now live. Thus, IAPI children are forced by circumstances to acquire English (or another language of their new motherland), and they do so in a context in which their own first languages have no use. For the first several months, communication is one of the most pressing issues in adoptive families. The motivation to acquire language is much more intense in international adoptees than in bilingual children from the immigrant families as IAPI children live in the monolingual (English only) total environment. Adoptive family is the primary source of patterns of proper English, while the same family cannot be a sustained source of the native language. Due to this situation, which is quite different from the immigrant families where a language other than English is the primary mode of communication, the native language of an adoptee quickly loses its functionality and personal meaning. At the same time, due to "survival" motivation, IAPI children master the communicative aspect of the English language more rapidly than their peers from immigrant families.

Language Attrition: Functional vs. Total

Language attrition in IAPI children is the process of losing their first (native for them) language. Language is a psychological function, and all functions exist only if they exercised: "use it or lose it" as the saying goes. If a language is not in use, it stagnates: does not develop, stays frozen at the level of entry to the new linguistic environment initially, and, finally, disappears for all practical purposes. There are two levels of language attrition: functional and total. Functional language attrition means that although a child may retain the remnants of the first language, particularly in receptive domain, this language cannot be used for its major functional operations like communication, behavior regulation, learning, and reasoning. Total language loss happens when no traces of it can be detected; the person does not comprehend even the most elementary communication, cannot produce any words, and repeats the phases from his former native language with distinct foreign accent and intonation.

Social/Communicative Language vs. Cognitive/Academic Language

Communicative language refers to the language skills needed for social interactions in everyday communication within a practical and familiar context. It includes basic skills in pronunciation, vocabulary, and grammar. It often includes a so-called sight vocabulary, which is the ability to read simple signs like "Exit," "No Smoking," etc. Communicative fluency is highly contextual and is supported by extralinguistic means, such as gestures, facial expressions, intonation, and body postures. This aspect of language seems to be acquired naturally and without formal schooling. A lively informal discussion of the latest baseball match at a family picnic table is an example of communicative language use.

Cognitive language refers to language as a tool of reasoning, a means of literacy, and a medium for academic learning. The mastery of cognitive language requires specific conceptual and semantic knowledge of the language itself. This language function emerges and becomes distinctive with formal schooling and developing literacy skills. Reading a scientific text about a volcanic eruption and writing an essay about warning signs of a possible volcanic eruption in a fifth-grade science project is an example of using cognitive/academic language.

Developmentally, communicative language forms first and serves as the base for cognitive language acquisition. The quality and quantity of a child's early communicative experience is crucial for forming the foundation of cognitive/academic language. Certain properties of cognitive language, such as grammar structures and lexicology patterns, are simply embedded into the psychological makeup of native speakers through frequent repetition when they were infants and toddlers, and their parents were talking to them or near them, or reading to them, or through TV or computers' games. Nothing is ever wasted; indeed, this information goes to a psychological storage vault and later is activated through the conscious efforts of schoolteachers and students themselves. In other words, children are predisposed to cognitive language mastery through their earlier experiences with the language: when a teacher introduces notions and concepts through language, the children evoke preexisting patterns, the absence of which may contribute to the failure in mastering reading and writing skills.

In children adopted after age five, the order of learning language skills is broken: upon arrival, they enter school and must learn understanding, speaking, reading, and writing skills of their new language simultaneously.

Language as Behavior Regulator

In the context of international adoption, this is an extremely important language function that explains many aspects of IAPI children's social/behavioral performance. Behavior regulation utility of language is responsible for the control and management of other people's actions, including modification of our own behavior. During silent monologues, we encourage ourselves, we explain, inspire, and justify the intentions. In the social milieu, we explain what we want; we demand, threaten, or beg and thus regulate the behavior of others: almost all of our external regulations are conducted via language. Slow language development plays a role in behavioral difficulties across the life span, demonstrating high comorbidity of language impairment with behavior problems (Van Daal, Verhoeven, & van Balkom, 2007). Children who are unable to communicate effectively may not have the necessary skills to negotiate or resolve conflict and may have difficulties understanding and relating to others. On the other hand, a number of studies pointed to positive associations between language mastery and pro-social and self-regulatory behavior (Spira & Fischel, 2005; Bolter & Cohen, 2007).

Vygotsky stated that cognitive and behavioral self-regulation is mastered through a process in which children learn their culture's symbols and thoughts, internalizing their caregivers' regulatory verbal input. Indeed, children who have verbal means to express their feelings and desires can better regulate their behaviors and the behaviors of others to confirm with the social expectations for their age. Those who have larger vocabularies, indicative of larger symbolic repertoires, have more mental tools to use in service of self-regulation. There is a body of research linking self-regulation and language skills (Ponitz, McClelland, Matthews, & Morrison, 2009). There are studies showing associations between delayed language and behavior problems. For example, observing preschool children with and without language delays in a classroom setting, Qi and Kaiser (2004) found that preschoolers with language delays more often acted aggressively and disruptively, and were less likely to initiate and engage pro-socially.

Language Development Before Adoption

A non-stimulating environment of early language development in IAPI children makes them a high-risk group for later language disorders and delays. Thus some of the most common notations in the orphanage-based medical records of children ages 3 and up are "delay in language development" and "speech and language disorder." Sometimes a specific diagnosis is indicated, such as *dysarthria* (faulty speech articulation). Sometimes no diagnosis is available, but speech and language remediations are mentioned as either provided or needed (Ladage, 2009).

In a book published in Moscow by a group of Russian psychologists (Dubrovina & Ruzskay, 1991), the authors describe what they call a "temporal delay in psychological development" as typical of children raised in orphanages due to a lack of stimulation in early childhood. They specifically point to delays in speech and language development. The common picture for many orphanage children in Russia at the age of 3 is incomprehensible vocalizations with only a few words and noticeable slowness in learning new words. At the age of 4, the same problem persists with attempts to use somewhat longer sentences, usually with faulty grammar. In one study described in the book, it was found that about 60% of all 2.5-year-olds in a Babies Home (orphanages for infants and toddlers—BG) had no expressive language at all, not a single word, just incomprehensible vocalizations. A year later, only a small percentage of a group of 106 3-and-a-half-year-old children used two-word sentences. The authors suggested that this situation is not only due to a severe lack of quality and quantity of verbal interaction between a child and an adult during the critical periods of language development, but mostly because of the very context of the communication.

Dubrovina and her colleagues made a following observation: they wrote that for babies in an orphanage, the goal of communication with an adult is physical contact and attention. Mutual object-related activity and cognitive learning activities are very limited, which has a detrimental impact on language development. In fact, a child does not need language to attract a smile, a hug, or a pat on the shoulder: for this, it is enough to approach an adult, touch her or pull her arm, and establish eye contact with her. It is when a child wants an adult's help and joint efforts in object- or person-related activity (e.g., to open a box to see what is inside, to turn the page to find a picture, or reading a book) that language emerges as a means of communication and regulation of behavior (Dubrovina, 1991, pp. 101–123).

According to Benilova (2014, p. 536), over half of all inmates of orphanages in Russia from ages 4 to 6 suffered from what she termed "systemic speech and language underdevelopment." The author described the following symptoms (translation is mine—BG):

Children with second and third degree of dysarthria . . . mixing morphological elements of language in chaotic and disorganized combinations out of logical laws of the mother tongue . . . children use a form of words regardless of the value that must be expressed in connection with the syntax. Another clear manifestation of verbal dys-ontogenesis is an inappropriate combination of pretexts and case forms. Agrammatism is the most stable and one of the main manifestations of the systemic underdevelopment of language.

Two researchers from Russia (Tumanova & Filicheva, 2017) noted that orphanage residents may have primary normal hearing and "conserved intellect" but still demonstrate difficulties with vocabulary, grammar, phonetics, and, as a consequence, limitations in communicative speech. The variability of the manifestations and severity of speech and language disorders are well above the incidents of the same disorders when compared to children raised in families.

Similarly, Asimina, Melpomeni, and Alexandra (2017) found that in Greek orphanages, children had significantly lower scores in the expressive language, receptive vocabulary, and narrative skills than children raised in families.

According to the most comprehensive research of the current orphanages (the St. Petersburg—USA Orphanage Research Team report, 2009), speech and language delays and disorders are the most consistent deficiency noted in orphanage-raised children. Having poorly developed their native languages, IAPI children face the challenge of learning a new language. It is a well-established fact that proficiency in the first language serves as a scaffold for successful learning of the second language. The first language forms the foundation upon which the second language acquisition will take place. The initial delay in the first language means that a less supportive foundation for English language learning exists. With a wide spectrum of different predictions of success in learning new language, the old finding—proficiency in first (native) language—still holds true (Krakow, Tao, & Roberts, 2005; Bardovi-Harlig & Stringer, 2010; Glennen, 2014, 2015).

Language Development After Adoption

The reported research findings in studies of language functioning for international adoptees after adoption could be confusing because of inconsistency and the wide variability of findings. It could be due to methodological differences, such as the use of direct assessment via standardized tests versus parent/teacher reports. This situation poses a question about which standards are appropriate and valid for the identification of language problems in IAPI children. The existing methods—the tests that were standardized on a population at large—may not be appropriate and valid for IAPI children because (from a strictly psychometric tenet) a comparison with peers in the standardization samples represents statistically improbable and unrealistic standards. Still a separate issue is the differentiation between language impairment and temporary difficulties in new language learning (Elleseff, 2013). In general, the results of the research on speech and language functioning of IAPI children are so divergent and conflicting that Glennen ends up with a call to better understand (Glennen, 2016, p. 148) *"who was assessed, what was measured, and the 'lens' used to view the results."* Unfortunately, after many years of international adoption on a large scale, we still do not know the prevalence and the nature of language problems IAPI children.

One common ground is that the majority of specialists consider IAPI children to be an "at risk" group for language development. The rate of referrals for speech and language services among IAPI children (after the English language became their only functional language) is statistically significantly above expectations for the population at large (Glennen, 2005; 2007a, 2007b; Eigsti, Weitzman, Schun, DeMarchena, & Casey, 2011; Gauthier & Genesee, 2011; Genesee, 2016). Even in children adopted from different countries before their second birthday and after living in adoptive families for at least two years, the rate of referral for speech and language services was from 22% to 35% (Mason & Narad, 2005; Glennen, 2005; Geren, Snedeker, & Ax, 2005; Francis, 2005). This is significantly higher than the 2% to 8% rate reported in the general preschool population, ages 3 through 6 (Glennen (2007a).

Several publications suggest that, while there are impressive advances in early language learning, delays may become noticeable when children reach school-age and must use their language to accomplish more complex academic and cognitive tasks (Dalen, 2001; Gindis, 2004; Goodman, 2013; Glennen, 2014, 2015). The "older" adoptees (adopted at preschool and school-age), showed impairments in language abilities, even after several years with the adoptive families and consistent exposure to a high level of English (Scott, Roberts, & Krakow, 2008; Hough & Kaczmarek, 2011; Scott et al., 2011). Thus, according to a Pearson (2010) study of 175 IAPI children adopted after the age of 3, about 25% of all children exhibited moderate to severe delay in comprehension of communicative language and 34% in production of communicative language after one year in adoptive homes. A study of adoptees who, by virtue of their early life experiences, vary significantly in their language abilities may illuminate links between language acquisition and adverse childhood experience. Thus Eigsti et al. (2011) proposed *"that exposure to chronic stress, operationalized as the duration of institutionalization, has specific neural effects on cognitive processes that are involved in language acquisition"* (p. 629).

Here is a real-life clinical case from my practice to illustrate the effects of traumatic social events on language issues in IAPI children.

Clinical Case: IAPI Children With No First Language

This nonfiction story started in a grim and dismal industrial city called Pavlodar in northern Kazakhstan, located near the southern border with the Russian Federation. After a single mother (ethnically a Slavic woman) was stripped of her maternal rights for drug and alcohol abuse combined with total neglect of her children, her two kids, a 3-year-old girl and a 5-year-old boy, were sent to a local orphanage. The city of Pavlodar's

Russian-speaking orphanages had no vacancies, and both kids were further transported to another orphanage in a rural, exclusively Kazakh-speaking area.

The kids found themselves in a situation where their nascent communicative Russian had no use. They had to start learning the Kazakh language, and as it always happens with language attrition, their Russian vanished. And according to the language acquisition rules, their Kazakh, shaped mostly by peers, came along, composed of limited and highly pragmatic vocabulary. Two years passed by. The boy turned 7 years old. When approving the list of first graders, the principal of the orphanage-based school stumbled upon a Russian surname—our siblings were the only ethnic Russians in the orphanage—and crossed them out. They didn't belong in the Kazakh school because the regulations required Russians to study both languages at the time, while one was sufficient for the Kazakh students.

The principal submitted a transfer request, and the boy and his sister went back to the city of Pavlodar. It didn't take long for teachers to find out that neither of them spoke Russian, already supplanted by the Kazakh oral language. All these educational misadventures were accompanied by constant teasing and bullying by their peers in the orphanages. In the Kazakh orphanage, the local kids beat them up as *dumb Russians*. In the mostly Russian-speaking city orphanage, the story mirrored itself: despite their Slavic appearance, the brother and sister spoke exclusively Kazakh and were treated badly by their Russian-speaking peers. The next two years were a struggle to pick up Russian.

By the time an American couple adopted the siblings, their Kazakh had diminished to the degree of near extinction, and their Russian became only barely functional. The boy was 9 years old and his sister 7. Together with the kids, the adoptive parents brought an English-Russian-Kazakh speaking nanny to the US, hired to help during the initial post-adoption period.

The new au pair, Irma, was an educated Kazakh woman in her late 20s who left her husband and daughter at home for the chance to make some money in America. Irma used to be an English teacher and had no difficulties with English or Russian, not to mention her native Kazakh. "Speak Kazakh and Russian to them," the adoptive parents instructed Irma. "It will be great if the children retain their languages."

Wealthy but uninvolved, the adoptive parents skipped the psychological screening of the kids and relied on the nanny-translator to solve all school issues. In September, the kids went to a public school—a regular class in an affluent New York suburban neighborhood. No one expected them to speak English right away, but after two semesters of English as a Second Language (ESL), unsuccessful despite attention in school and tutoring at home, their teachers asked for an assessment. "We need to make sure they aren't learning disabled. Kazakhstan, you said? But aren't they ethnically Russian? So, we need a Russian-speaking bilingual psychologist," the school authority reasoned. That's how the children, accompanied by their nanny, ended up in my office.

After a brief verbal exchange, I found myself at a "dead end" language-wise. Seemingly normal and physically well developed, the 10-year-old boy and his 8-year-old sister had enough language for neither communication, nor behavior regulation, nor cognitive reasoning! All they understood was a primitive receptive Russian—sit down, stand up—not nearly enough for an assessment. Their expressive Russian consisted of a limited misarticulated vocabulary, framed into the severely distorted grammar normally found in 2-year-olds. I switched to English only to be discouraged again; its functional level didn't differ much from the Russian, which was very unusual after almost 15 months of direct exposure and ESL instructions.

"How's their Kazakh?" I asked Irma.

"Rudimentary, not really functional," confirmed the au pair.

"How do they talk to their parents and teachers?"

"I help translate at home and in school."

"From what language?"

"They use their own jargon, a jumble of Russian, Kazakh, and English. No grammar or sentence structure, more like a baby talk. I kind of understand it now."

"What about reading and writing in English?" I asked.

"No progress. We got stuck with printing words from a sample. They do not understand the very concept that letters represent sounds."

I had in front of me two physically and sensory intact children, who, due to the bizarre social circumstances of development, were deprived of the most basic human ability: use of language. In my examination, I had to rely more on a nonverbal assessment with all its limitations. The results showed normal cognitive potential and visual-based reasoning within the age norms, although on the lower side. Under normal circumstances, they could attend school, but the lack of the magic medium to pass the material along deemed the brother and sister severely learning impaired. They needed special education placement and programming with an emphasis on English. Their bi- and trilingualism was to be discarded. Regardless of their age, they had to start from the preschool level in their language development.

Although this example with no-first-language siblings may appear to be a rare deviation, it reflects the influential social factor in the language development of IAPI children.

In the US, internationally adopted children are entitled to a school-related assessment in their native language under the Individuals with

Disabilities Education Act (IDEA). This assessment must take place within the first weeks of their arrival. Due to a fast-moving, first-language attrition, each week of delay rapidly narrows the window of opportunity for an accurate and informative evaluation in the native language. The fact that IAPI children have a high rate of speech and language problems underscores the need to differentiate between the temporary difficulties in second-language learning and a genuine language disorder or delay. Making a differential diagnosis is a great challenge for an educational diagnostician, and the key to it is a speech and language evaluation in the first language while it still exists.

Let us consider a rather typical situation with a parent in my office, describing her 7-year, 4-month-old daughter, adopted at the age of 6 years and 2 months. The parent reported that the child, who lost her native Ukrainian for all practical purposes, in English

- depends on gesturing to be understood;
- systematically confuses tenses, personal pronouns, and plurals;
- omits parts of sentences;
- substitutes, omits, distorts, and reverses sounds in words;
- has difficulty in using multiple meaning words;
- often fails to discriminate between words that look or sound alike;
- demonstrates delayed responses when questioned;
- uses nonspecific referential terms (that, this, thing, stuff) instead of the needed precise labels; and
- lacks in comprehension and sometimes gives irrelevant responses.

The adoptive parent presented this list of language difficulties to the girl's second-grade teacher. The teacher agreed: "I have observed pretty much the same, but this is normal for a child of her age who is just learning a new language. Leave her alone, and in a year or two she will be just fine." In some way, the teacher may be right: these symptoms are characteristic of the process of new language learning, but these could be symptoms of heavy language problems. If similar patterns were found in the child's first language (that had disappeared by the time of the parent-teacher conference), then we could have claimed with certainty a genuine language disorder, not a passing difficulty in new language learning. With the closure of this narrow window of opportunity to find the problems early on, proper identification and remediation of the issues is delayed for a year or two, sometimes irreversibly. Most parents and teachers are simply unable to differentiate between language disorder/delay (for which speech/language therapy is needed) and a typical language acquisition process for which time is required and extensive ESL instruction is in order. Time may provide the answer, but it also presents the risk that a child will continue to fall behind as the school and the parents are "waiting." A speech and language pathologist, who administers the assessment, must be well versed in the concept of language attrition and learn about the major signs and indicators of this process.

First-Language Attrition

One of the most impressive descriptions of native language loss as a personal traumatic experience was provided by William Shakespeare. In his *Richard II* masterpiece, Thomas Mowbray Duke of Norfolk, thinking about his exile, fears most of all that his mother tongue will be without use and vanish:

> *The language I have learn'd these forty years,*
> *My native English, now I must forego*
> *[. . .]*
> *I am too old to fawn upon a nurse,*
> *Too far in years to be a pupil now:*
> *What is thy sentence then but speechless death,*
> *Which robs my tongue from breathing native breath?*

With only a few exceptions, the vast majority of IAPI children adopted by monolingual English-speaking families are going through language attrition—loss of their native language. The swiftness with which IAPI children lose their native tongue and the profound nature of that loss are truly amazing.

The phenomenon of language attrition is not new or unusual: it is often observed in immigrants of all ages (Fillmore, 1991; Schmid, 2002; Bylund, 2009). It was mostly studied in immigrant children whose families continued to speak in their native language. Although first-language attrition is widespread in children from these families, international adoptees differ from children from immigrant families, as they have diverse causes and distinctive dynamics of their native language loss.

First, in IAPI children, we see the abrupt and immediate cessation of access to the native language with the exact date when it started—the day when the newly adopted child landed on American soil. Second, the motivation to learn the new language in IAPI children is equal to the survival drive—not the same educational goals as in immigrant children who continue to use their native language in their families and often in their communities. Third, the base of native language is so weak that the attrition process encounters little resistance.

The study of linguistic mechanisms of first-language attrition in international adoptees is still in its embryonic phase. From the limited research in this domain, it appears that the pattern of language attrition in international adoptees follows the general pattern found in children from immigrant families: the literacy skills in their native language disappear first, followed by expressive language, and then receptive language. The psychoeducational consequences of first language loss in this population have been studied even less, although these issues have major practical significance.

There are four important aspects of language attrition recognized and investigated by contemporary scientists: neurological (brain plasticity, neuron-based activation, and inhibition thresholds), cognitive (memory, aptitude, and literacy), emotional/motivational (feelings and attitudes), and cultural/social (the cultural context and social value) (Schmid, 2004, 2012; Levy, McVeigh, Marful, & Anderson, 2007; Linck, Judith, Kroll, & Sunderman, 2009; Schmid & Dusseldorp, 2010; Schmid, Köpke, & de Bot, 2012, Schmid & Köpke, 2013). None of these factors alone is responsible for the language attrition; therefore, a multifaceted research approach to language attrition is the most productive way. Indeed, all listed factors form a system that makes sense only if contemplated as a whole. Moreover, language attrition, although obviously an individual phenomenon, cannot be understood outside of the social context: it happens at the intersection of individual capacity and social factors (Köpke, 2007; Schmitt, 2010).

Functional language loss means that a language cannot be used for its major applications: communication, behavior regulation, learning, reasoning, and other cognitive operations. Here is an extract from a bilingual assessment of a child who was adopted from Russia at the age of 11 years and 3 months, and was tested 3 years later, at the age of 14 years and 2 months.

> It is this examiner's conclusion that at the time of this assessment, Pavel does not have functional communicative skills in the Russian language. In terms of his receptive language, Pavel barely understood simple commands accompanied by a gesture (e.g., "Move the chair closer to the desk"). He responded to short, context-embedded, concrete instructions on the level expected of a three-year-old native speaker. His retrieval fluency and naming vocabulary in Russian were comparable to a child no older than three. In terms of expressive language, Pavel is able to produce only several words in Russian on his own, all these words with distorted pronunciation (foreign accent). I tried to extract any communication in Russian from Pavel, but what I was able to elicit did not exceed a single word. Being asked to repeat simple (from two to three words) sentences after the examiner, Pavel used the English language intonation patterns in Russian grammatical constructions. Being asked to conjugate nouns, verbs, and numerals in the Russian language, he distorted them like a foreigner in the beginning stage of learning language. Responding to the Picture Vocabulary subtests from the Bilingual Verbal Ability Tests (BVAT), Russian Form, Pavel was able to name only nine objects in Russian and in almost half of all cases he was able to name

the function but not the exact label of the object. Thus, pointing to the picture of a telephone he said "zvonit," which means "to ring." When he was able to name an object in Russian, he expressed such joy (smiling and clapping with his hands) that it was obvious he had tried his best to name the pictures in Russian but could not remember much in his first language. Pavel cannot read or write in Russian and was able to name correctly only three letters in the Russian alphabet.

Total language loss may be diagnosed when no traces of language are detectable; the child does not comprehend even the most elementary communication, cannot produce any words, repeats the phrases in his former native language with a foreign accent and intonation, and cannot distinguish his former native tongue from verbalization in any other language.

Impressive description of total language loss was presented in research published by Pallier and his colleagues in France (Pallier, Ventureyra, & Yoo, 2004). Young adults, all adopted from South Korea as preschool and school-aged children (ages 3 through 9), were subjected to a rather sophisticated set of neurological, psychological, and linguistic tests in their early 20s. The finding was that there was no trace of the birth language, not even recognition of elementary bits of language, and no differential brain activation when the participants were exposed auditorily to spoken Korean as opposed to other, unknown languages. The cortical regions that showed greater response to the known language, French, were similar in the adopted subjects and in the French monolingual controls. Pallier and his coauthors suggested that the total cessation of first language was responsible for this situation. The researchers suggested that the presence of the first language (all children were monolingual in Korean at the time of adoption) acted as a block to French language acquisition and that when all contacts to Korean language were terminated, the neural network was "reset" to allow these children to become monolingual again, this time in French. Functional MRI studies of adults who were internationally adopted as children found that adult adoptees no longer recognized phonology of their first language in spite of the fact that some of them were adopted at the age 7 to 9 years. A positive aspect of first-language attrition was stressed in the Pallier et al. (2004) publication: according to the authors, attrition of the birth language in IAPI children "cleans the slate" and allows for a full acquisition of the adopted language.

Many other investigations tried to challenge Pallier's conclusions by attempting to establish whether adoptees might have a relearning benefit when they make efforts to acquire their birth language again later in life (Hyltenstam, Bylund, Abrahamsson, & Park, 2009; Schmitt, 2010). So far, the findings from these investigations were ambiguous and did not support the theory of total language replacement or the theory of retention as a relearning benefit. This is clearly one of the areas of investigation that will be of crucial importance to language attrition studies in the coming years.

I conducted my own experiment related to native language recognition, which is briefly described here.

Two women (ages 25 and 61, mother and daughter), read a text—about 400 words—half in Russian and half in Ukrainian (eastern Ukraine dialect). The text was read as one piece without pause. Please note that both languages belong to the same group of Slavic languages and have overwhelming likenesses, particularly grammatically and syntactically, but are substantially different in intonation (the melodic pattern of an utterance) and vocabulary.

The question was, Is this text in the same or different languages?

Twelve monolingual, English-only students (8 females and 4 males ages 19 to 27) from Touro College in New York listened to the tape individually. None of the listeners knew Ukrainian or Russian languages. Only 2 out of 12 were able to say that the text was, likely, in two different but similar languages because the intonation was different. When the same text was given to seven native Russian-speaking adults, all seven said that the tape was recorded in two languages, Russian and Ukrainian. The differentiation of two languages was made instantly, and no one among the participants experienced any doubts.

Finally, the same test was given individually to 16 IAPI children. All were adopted from Russia between ages 5 and 9, being at that time monolingual Russian individuals. All were tested after living in the US from 4 and 6 years. Seven out of 16 were able to say that the text was recorded in Russian; others were not able even to recognize the language. And none was able to distinguish between the Russian and Ukrainian languages! The language attrition was so deep and comprehensive that recognition of the differences, so obvious for any native Russian speaker, was impossible for the now totally monolingual, English-only adolescents adopted mostly at school-age.

One of the most well-known explanations of language attrition is the "neural plasticity theory": early neurocognitive traces of the birth language are erased when they are no longer useful, thereby creating a neurocognitive state, akin to the state in which babies are typically in when learning their first language. Genesee (2016) provides a review of evidences for and against this theory.

Time Frames of Language Attrition

In many parent surveys and some research publications (Wong-Fillmore, 1991; Schmid, 2007; Pearson, 2008), the time frames of functional language attrition are tied to the age at adoption: the younger the child, the faster the attrition is completed. Our own study of more than 700 children, ages 3 to 17, adopted from overseas orphanages all over the world between 1990 and 2017 revealed the relatively consistent pattern of

Table 4.1 Time Frames of Language Attrition for IAPI Children

Age at Adoption	Expressive Language	Receptive Language
3.6–4.0	7–12 weeks	11–15 weeks
4.0–6.0	2–3 months	3–5 months
6.0–7.0	2–3 months	Up to 6 months
7.0–9.0	3–6 months	Up to 9–12 months

the time frames of functional language attrition for different age groups. Native languages in this study were Russian, Ukrainian, Chinese, Spanish, and Amharic (an official language in Ethiopia).

The youngest group for which we have clinical data is 3 years 6 months to 4 years. Expressive language usually is rather weak in this age group, often with pronounced articulation difficulties, immature word usage, and faulty grammar in short sentences. In the situation of full English language immersion, it takes these children 7 to 12 weeks to reduce their expressive language to practically a nonfunctional state. Their receptive language may stay several weeks longer, but it is barely functional, even in familiar situations with the support of gestures, voice tone, and other nonlinguistic means of communication.

For 6- to 9-year-old IAPI children, the same process of losing language functionality may take up to six months, with the erosion of the language increasing with each passing week of living in an English-only environment. It may take longer for older adoptees, particularly in sibling groups.

There is a notion that literacy skills (reading and writing) may prevent or slow down attrition, and this is hard to object to because it sounds reasonable. At the beginning of our clinical work with older IAPI children, our group of specialists at the BGCenter thought the same way: the children who were able to read and write in their native language should resist language attrition longer. After all, literacy means certain cognitive organization and structure, and through literacy, reading first of all, children can maintain the use of their first language as a purposeful psychological function. As Köpke (2007) wrote, *"Less attrition is to be expected in subjects who have had the opportunity to become literate in the L1, especially if they frequently use that skill"* (p. 3). The last part of this statement is crucial—indeed, if a person practices reading often in the first language, the attrition may be slowed down and probably prevented. Unfortunately, this is not the case with the majority of international adoptees. Isolated from the everyday environment, initial literacy skills do not survive and don't help to preserve the language. With constant use and the intrinsic motivation to keep the literacy skills, initial literary skills may help suspend the attrition, but if idle, they prove immaterial and don't prevent the loss. Once the process of attrition starts, literacy becomes its first casualty, followed by expressive skills, and finally the receptive language loss. The principle here is "last in, first out": the last acquired skill disappears first. In short, our clinical data did not support the notion of literacy as a protective factor against first-language attrition: children with elementary literacy skills in their native languages showed the same speed of attrition as illiterate peers.

In terms of the English language learning, all IAPI children go through a so-called transitional period that starts when the child steps on American land and ends with having English as the only functional language. The end of the transitional period does not mean the mastery of new language at the age-expected level, but rather that English is now the child's native language as defined by the law.

The definition of native language in IDEA (Part B Code of Federal Regulations: CFR §300.19) is very clear:

(a) As used in this part, the term native language, if used with reference to an individual of limited English proficiency, means the following:

   (1) The language normally used by that individual, or, in the case of a child, the language normally used by the parents of the child, except as provided in paragraph (a)(2) of this section.

   (2) In all direct contact with a child (including evaluation of the child), the language normally used by the child in the home or learning environment.

In the situation of an internationally adopted child, in contrast to any other group of English language learners, English satisfies both paragraphs (1) and (2) of the code. Therefore, even though the IAPI child is an individual of Limited English Proficiency (LEP), his or her native language should be defined as English.

Causes of Rapid Native Language Loss in IAPI Children

Kopke (2007) listed the following brain processors that involved in language attrition: 1) plasticity (dependent on the age at onset of attrition and new language learning), 2) activation, 3) inhibition (both are linked to frequency of competing language use), and 4) the subcortical involvement (a function of emotional implications of the first or second language). In IAPI children, a radical change in the linguistic environment requires quick adjustment to the new language situation: learning the adoptive family language on top of not using the first one. According to the concept of brain plasticity, the younger the subject is, the more effective learning takes place and the easier the erosion and disappearance of the first language (Nelson, 2002; Schmid & Kopke, 2013).

Activation and inhibition are two sides of the same process: the individuals who make little use of a language suffer more from attrition than speakers who use the language more frequently. The quality of use, or type of contact, is equally important. Both processes, learning English and losing the native language, are the by-products of participation in a range of activities in the given social groups, such as family, school, community, peers, and social media. Linguistic isolation that leads to disappearing language as the most important social facility has a lasting psychological impact. In addition to age and the frequency of the native language use while living in an English-only environment, the following factors are known to facilitate first-language attrition in IAPI children:

- Initial low level of first-language skills: incomplete acquisition of the first language facilitates its rapid attrition (Gindis, 1999a, 2004, 2005; Elleseff, 2011).
- Individual differences: certain neurological mechanisms, cognitive qualities, and internal motivations of a person: no practical need in keeping the language as a means of social interaction results in a lack of internal motivation to sustain the first language.
- Social interaction factor: preadolescents and adolescents in particular are oriented toward the conditions of acceptance by their peers to "mix with the crowd," be like others, and conform to the peer group's approved norms and expectations. But any foreign language is a marker of being "external" and different, and therefore is not a needed skill in the perception of an IAPI adolescent. School-aged children are prone to language attrition, as they are strongly motivated to integrate into the new language environment.
- Trauma-related factor: this rather significant reason for a rapid loss of the first language, particularly in older adoptees, often stays under the scientific radar. The adverse trauma-related personal feelings and attitudes toward a native language are crucial to its maintenance or attrition. This factor deserves our special attention due to its specificity for IAPI as seen from the following:

The date upon arrival in the new motherland constitutes a natural boundary, separating two universes: pre-adoption and post-adoption. For an IAPI child, every aspect of life has changed after adoption: the food, the clothes, the language, the social milieu, etc., even something as personal as one's name is often changed. Language remains a single thread connecting adoptees to the past, which is not a "paradise lost," but for some may be nightmarish memories of neglect, hunger, and abuse. The language is often the only connection with those days of misery and suffering, and it needs to disappear as soon as possible because pain and sorrow are not the luggage one wishes to carry into the future. Language, as the obvious link to the past, is to be severed as soon as possible to preserve the mental health of the language carrier.

Research (Isurin, 2000; Nicoladis & Grabois, 2002; Pavlenko, 2005; Gardner, 2010) suggests that strong emotional events may have serious consequences for language attrition. Emotion is most likely a key factor in any case of attrition, and it may play an even bigger role in language attrition than in language acquisition (Kouritzin, 1999). It is predictable that native language attrition would likely occur faster in cases in which the first language is strongly rejected as a connecting link to the traumatic past. In other words, attrition is facilitated by the native language rejection as the result of trauma. Thus M. Schmidt in her book *First Language Attrition, Use and Maintenance* (2002) was among the first ones who closely connected language attrition to negative emotional reaction toward a first language. From her analysis of the morpho-syntactic features of the German language and other purely linguistic phenomena, the intensity of the persecution was the decisive factor in language attrition, particularly in younger refugees from the Nazi regime.

Experts in the treatment of disorders stemming from traumatic experiences have long since identified language, even a mere sound of language, as a potential trigger of post-traumatic stress disorder (Kouritzin, 1999). This should not be a surprise, because language is the single prevailing representation of a person's individual life history: it is the compelling link between the present and the past, and it is the most prominent "marker" of belonging to a certain ethnic and cultural group.

IAPI children, especially those adopted after the preschool years, have memories of their traumatic past. For many adoptees, their native language is a constant reminder of their suffering—an experience most of them are trying to overcome. They want to blend as soon as possible with their new peers, to look the same, to act the same, and to speak the same language. The easiest way to cut ties with the past and to identify with the present is to destroy the obvious link: the language. Forgetting the language seems to have a positive therapeutic value for many IAPI children, while externally imposed demands to keep the language may traumatize them. Emotional feelings and cognitive attitudes influence the process of first-language disappearance and second-language acquisition. Thus adoptive parents presenting positive feelings toward the new language community can facilitate learning, resulting in higher proficiency levels (Gardner, 2010). The same is true in relation to first-language attrition: negative attitude and adverse emotional reaction to their mother tongue facilitates native language attrition.

Rejection of the first language is common in adopted children, making them different from children who emigrate as part of a non-English-speaking family where many, not all, routinely become comfortably bilingual with English as their dominant language. Not so with former residents of orphanages: as part of the process of solidifying their new identities, they almost always consciously or subconsciously discard their first language.

Here is what an adoptive parent wrote in his referral letter to our office:

It's sad in many ways, but clearly, my 7-year-old child wants nothing to do with the Spanish language or Guatemala itself. In fact, he gets hysterical if we call him by his birth name, Miguel, which we ended up keeping for his middle name. He associates it with his other life, a life that he is doing everything he can to forget. And this is a little boy with no attachment issues whatsoever, who was, in our opinion, well-cared for by the orphanage staff, and who seemed pretty happy all in all when we met him. I don't think we'll ever know exactly the underlying issues, and I imagine one day he will want information about his previous life, but for now, at least, he has no interest whatsoever in anything related to his native country and his first language.

Patterns of First-Language Attrition in IAPI Children

A language is not a uniform phenomenon, and its components resist attrition with various degrees of success. Different language elements—pragmatical, phonological, lexical, and morpho-syntactic—may reveal different degrees of attrition dynamic (Bardovi-Harlig & Stringer, 2010). According to some sources (Pierce, Klein, Chen, Delcenserie, & Genesee, 2014), the phonological elements of language are retained longer than later-acquired elements such as morpho-syntax or grammar. In my clinical experience, just the opposite was observed: at the beginning stages of native language attrition, I noted the loss of the specifics for Russian and Ukrainian languages intonation, stresses, and voice pitch patterns, particularly in connected speech. I agree with Pavlenko (2005, 2014), who wrote that language phonology plays a significant role in attrition: first-language attrition arises from suppression of the native language phonology during second-language usage. It is agreed upon that the vocabulary of the first language is affected before the grammatical and syntactical competency is lost (Schmid & Dusseldorp, 2010). As soon as a child absorbs a name of an object in English, the equivalent in the native language fades away and a retrieval of this word in the first language requires special effort in memory self-regulation. As a Russian poet O. Mandelstam once expressed it (cited by L. Vygotsky in his Thought and Language, 1986, p. 210),

The word I forgot
Which once I wished to say
And voiceless thought
Returns to shadows' chamber

As soon as the word in the second language is firmly established, its equivalent in the first language steps into the "shadows' chamber" and after this vanishes for good, and its loss becomes irreversible.

A detailed analysis of first-language vocabulary decline by children whose native language input effectively ceased after their immersion into the English environment was presented in the work of Isurin (2000). This data analysis was based on the results of picture naming tasks and reaction time measurements. Three groups of words showed high vulnerability to forgetting: high frequency words, cognates, and semantically convergent pairs (pairs of words lexically distinguished in English but nondistinguished in the first language). Isurin stated that fast forgetting of these lexical items in the first language was related to the acquisition of their equivalents in the English language. The comparison of noun versus verb retention/acquisition suggested that there might be a delay in the first-language verb forgetting and the English-language verb acquisition at the early stage of an extensive exposure to the second language (Isurin, 2000).

Rapid weakening of vocabulary in the first language was observed at the BGCenter using the Bilingual Verbal Ability Test, Normative Update in three languages: Russian, Chinese, and Spanish (Gindis, 1999b, 2004). We used three tests of oral language proficiency from the BVAT: picture vocabulary, oral vocabulary (synonyms/antonyms), and verbal analogies, as well as informal assessment in spontaneous, unprompted, and improvised conversations. We came to the conclusion that grammatical attrition comes next after the loss of vocabulary in the language erosion and signifies structural disintegration of the first language due to interference from English. The overall conclusion regarding the prevailing pattern of first-language attrition in IAPI children was as follows: phonological attrition, including a foreign language intonation, starts the process of wearing away the first language, vocabulary, and, almost simultaneously, grammatical structure.

In IAPI school-aged children, cross-linguistic patterns of transfer and interference affect the transition from one dominant language to another. For example, a "phonetic spelling" pattern, which is typical for students with a background in Slavic languages (Russian, Ukrainian, Polish, etc.), interferes with spelling in English. Indeed, the Russian/Ukrainian/Polish languages are phonetic languages: written words are close in writing structure to sounded-out words, with a grapheme-phoneme direct correlation reaching over 90%. I know from the clinical (and personal) experience that "phonetic spelling" is an "overlearned" skill. The habit of writing by "sounding out" still remains a firm feature of international adoptees age 8 and older, as their mental setup interferes with their spelling skills in English. These students are to be taught and trained to relinquish the very idea of phonemic spelling in English, where grapheme-phoneme correspondence is minimal (e.g., the word "daughter" has eight letters and only four sounds).

Consequences of Rapid First-Language Loss

The overall toll paid for the abrupt loss of the first language depends on the child's age and a host of individual differences. First and foremost, from psychological and educational perspectives, abrupt attrition of the first language is no less than an interruption in language development, when rapid attrition of the first language prevents the transfer of basic linguistic skills from one language to the other. For some IAPI children, abrupt first-language loss may intensify cognitive weaknesses and contribute to a cumulative cognitive deficit (see the next chapter for discussion). Further, language is a powerful tool for regulation of behavior, and when this tool is taken away abruptly, a set of inappropriate, regressive, immature, or clearly maladaptive behaviors can be observed.

It is important to understand from pedagogical, remedial, and psychological perspectives that the tempo of losing and replacing language does not coincide with time: losing a language occurs faster than mastering a new one. But the demand for major language applications— communication, behavior regulation, learning, and cognitive operations— remains as strong as ever. Problems with language are likely to have a cascade of effects on academic and socioemotional functioning, which is when a rapid language attrition becomes a clearly trauma-producing factor, calling for a systematic and appropriate help.

An abrupt first-language attrition in IAPI children leads to behavior dysregulation: having a major tool of self-regulation diminished in effectiveness, they deteriorate in their behavior. A 6-year-old child in the first several weeks in the adoptive home may demonstrate temper tantrums, acting out, and other behaviors, usually expected from a 3-year-old. In some children, this "linguistic gap" may lead to a period of "communication regression," such as pointing and gesturing or "functional mutism," when no language is used for some time, as reported by many parents and professionals. Moreover, for months to come, parents are limited in their ability to regulate IAPI child's behavior as they otherwise do for a child for whom language is a customary instrument of interpersonal interaction.

Paradoxically, the more language-advanced an IAPI child is at the time of adoption, the more he or she suffers from losing the ability to use language as a tool of social "transactions." Those who had functional verbal skills and a leader status in their orphanages may experience a kind of a shock with losing the ability to control the world with language skills. In order to regain their status, to continue to attract attention, to control and manipulate their environment, they may turn to a regressed and clearly maladaptive behavior. Girls may become withdrawn and refuse to learn the new language; boys may show a lot of sudden outrage and act out. After mastering the basics of communication, they can resume more appropriate behavior.

For school-aged IAPI children, rapid attrition of the first language before the English language develops presents a significant educational challenge (Meese, 2002; Glennen, 2002, 2005; Gindis, 2005). It is manifested in numerous learning problems, showcasing cognitive weaknesses (e.g., vanishing of basic cognitive skills, such as patterning, sequencing, discriminating, etc.), interruption in overall language development, and amplifying emotional and behavioral issues to the extreme. This leads to numerous social and academic problems that ought to be addressed by educators and adoptive parents if the role of language as a regulator of behavior is properly understood.

Learning English: Social/Communicative Versus Cognitive/Academic Language Acquisition

Eventually, all IAPI children—some sooner, some later—learn to communicate in English and master literacy skills to different degrees. Basically, the pattern of English-language learning in international adoptees is the same as in other "circumstantial" English-language learners: the communicative aspect of the language is acquired first and the cognitive/academic aspect later. However, the time frame and overall dynamic of English-language learning is quite different in IAPI children compared to the offspring of immigrant families.

While according to some researchers (Collier, 1989; Cummins, 1996, 2000), it takes a school-aged (6 through 17) immigrant child about two years to reach a native speaker's proficiency in communicative English, this is not the case with international adoptees. According to parents' surveys and research data (Clauss & Baxter, 1997; Dalen, 2001; Glennen, 2002), as well as the published clinical experience (Gindis, 1998, 1999a, 2004), a fully functional communicative fluency is usually achieved by international adoptees of preschool and school-age (ages 5 and up) within the first 12 to 18 months of their lives in their new country. Depending on the age and individual differences, there are variations, but the overall trend is that communicative fluency comes into existence much faster in a situation of total language assimilation versus a bilingual situation with a language other than English at home. It is a strong urge with survival overtones that determines the speed of communicative English-language learning for international adoptees. This is not the case with the children from immigrant families, who do not necessarily use their second language outside of school.

According to the published research, it takes a school-aged immigrant child five to seven years to develop cognitive/academic English language comparable to the level of a native speaker of the same age (Collier, 1989; Cummins, 1996, 2000; Collier & Thomas, 1989, 2002). The time frame of five to seven years attributed to bilingual children for acquiring cognitive/academic English may or may not be applicable to internationally adopted children: currently, no reliable data exists. What we do know is that certain aspects of academic/cognitive language, such as vocabulary and basic grammar structure, are formed faster than others, such as conceptual language knowledge, comprehension of words with multiple meanings, or mastery of writing/reading skills (Desmarais, Roeber, Smith, & Pollak, 2012).

Thomas and Collier (2002) analyzed the data for more than 700,000 students across the US from 1996 to 2001. Note that internationally adopted children were not included in the pool of those immigrant children as a separate category. In general, the authors confirmed previous studies that typical immigrants with two to five years of on-grade-level, home-country schooling take five to seven years to reach the 50th normal curve equivalent (NCE) of what an average student would achieve at that grade level in English. What is important for us is that the authors indicated that there is a category of "disadvantaged" young immigrants, the majority of whom do not ever make it to the 50th NCE if they have some or all of the following characteristics:

- Interrupted education with less than two years of schooling in the home country
- History of trauma (war, severe neglect of basic physical needs, deprivation, torture, assault, persecution)
- Parent illiteracy and lack of support for standard English literacy in the home

The first and second characteristics apply also to the majority of IAPI children. On the other hand, the IAPI children have powerful facilitators in their parents, who are typically native English speakers, well-educated, and highly motivated to educate their children. This factor is their great advantage compared to typical immigrant children.

The fact, broadly recognized and confirmed in numerous publications, is that the cognitive/academic aspect of a new language, sometimes called CALP (cognitive/academic language proficiency), requires more time to attain, presents significant difficulty, and causes academic problems for IAPI children (Pearson, 2001, 2005; Glennen, 2014, 2015, 2016). A deficiency in cognitive/academic aspect of language leads to learning difficulties that may persist, failing to match the comprehensive and relentless efforts of both adoptive parents and educational professionals.

Cognitive/academic language competence has a strong cultural overtone: such images as Donald Duck or Dennis the Menace, or a tune from the movie Cinderella are intimate parts of native-speakers' language competency, what is called in cultural psychology as "shared meaning" (Vygotsky, 1934/1986). The lack of these subtle overtones and the lack of commonly shared knowledge of tales, rhythms, songs, stories, cartoons, etc., may impede the language competence of those born and raised outside mainstream America. Language mediates social interaction, and those who are less able to understand the subtle meaning conveyed by language may be less ready for age-appropriate social experiences.

For many months, IAPI children adopted at preschool age and older tend to understand the meaning of the English words very literally. Parents testified,

> *One evening early on, after a particularly insane dinner, I held up my thumb and forefinger about an inch apart and exclaimed, "I am this close to the edge, and when I go, it won't be fun!" My 7-year daughter, adopted at age 5, hopped out of her seat, came over and hugged me saying, "It's OK, Mama. I go with you!"*
>
> *Nina was at home for about two years . . . we were leaving to go somewhere. I looked at her and said, "OK, let's hit the road." She replied, "Oh no . . . that hurts." I realized she assumed I meant literally go out and hit the road surface.*
>
> *I still remember when 6-year-old Danny (home about 20 months) came unglued when I told him that on his birthday, I was going to race him on the scooter and BEAT him around the entire block! "No, Mama . . . please don't beat me! I will be good. You can win . . . you can have my cake!"*

Adoptive parents of an IAPI child are usually amazed and pleased by their child's progress in mastering basic communication skills and see no apparent reason to worry about language development. However, as early as first grade, problems often emerge. Here is a typical situation described by adoptive parents in their referral letter to BGCenter:

> *Maria joined our family at the age of 3 years and 4 months after living all her life in orphanage in Guatemala. As a preschooler, she developed great skill in speaking and understanding the English language. At the age of 5, she started kindergarten, and at that time, no one could distinguish her language from that of her peers born in this country. But her first-grade teacher observed that Maria had problems with remembering lengthy directions and answering many "why" questions. Maria had difficulties with understanding stories not related to her immediate experience. In the second grade, her reading problems emerged. However, nothing was done, and by the middle of the third grade, Maria's academic problems consolidated to the extent that a team of school professionals evaluated her. Maria was found to have normal IQ, but her reading and writing skills were well below her grade level. Her comprehension of oral academic instructions is strikingly below expectations for her age. . . . Are these still language issues?*

Unfortunately, neither teachers nor parents realize that communicative fluency in adopted children in many cases is not directly transferable into cognitive language mastery, resulting in reading and writing problems years after being adopted. The child's conversational proficiency in English is not enough to ensure the mastery of the English language needed for age-appropriate academic functioning.

A big question is why some adopted children suffer from a cognitive language deficit, while others in the same age group are able to master it successfully. More focused studies are needed, but practical experience shows at least three factors: age of adoption, individual differences of the child, and scaffolding received in the family and school. The overall findings are as follows:

- Conversational proficiency in a new language is not enough to ensure cognitive-academic mastery of the language.
- The time needed for communicative fluency proficiency is different than the time for cognitive/academic language mastery.
- The dynamics of language acquisition in internationally adopted and immigrant children is similar to that of two balls released at the top of a hill and rolling downhill. The heavier one accelerates faster, but in the end, when the slope levels, the lighter ball catches up and goes further. Adoptees follow the pattern of the heavier ball: getting ahead of immigrants, they master the communicative language much sooner, as it is a survival skill for them, but then they slow down and go through more trouble when it comes to the cognitive/academic language. One of the reasons for such difference is the abrupt attrition of the native tongue. Instead of building upon the existing linguistic foundation as immigrants do, adopted children must retreat and start learning cognitive-academic language from the very beginning. It is probably true that abrupt first-language attrition may give an advantage in mastering communicative language, but it turns into a handicap later in learning cognitive/academic language.

English-Language Learners

From the social/cultural and educational perspectives, IAPI children belong to a large, mixed, and constantly changing group of the population called English-language learners (ELL). This category of students consists mostly of children who were born outside of the US and arrived in the country with their families, or who were born to a language minority group here in the US and until school did not have much exposure to the English language. Most importantly, these children continue to use their first language in their families and often in their neighborhood. The majority of them are bilingual with one dominant language. Internationally adopted children, though a part of this diverse group, differ from the rest of the ELL classmates in many respects discussed earlier.

At present, ESL instructions is a mandatory program for every non-English-speaking child who enters the public school system in the US (Title VI of the Civil Rights Act of 1964, US Department of Education[1]). IAPI children are automatically eligible for this educational service; however, their situation is radically different from that of traditional "limited English proficiency" students. Indeed, from the moment of the adoption, international adoptees live in monolingual (English only) families, not in families where an "other-than-English" language is used. Actually, we have a unique situation when students eligible for ESL have the English language as their sole home language! This changes the overall context of second-language acquisition and brings a possibility of enrichment at home and more active parental involvement in the process of new language learning. Probably for the first time in the history of ESL instruction, parents may act as teachers of and "language role models" for their children, with a home "follow-up component" of the classroom instruction possible. No wonder many adoptive parents demand that the ESL instruction for international adoptees be modified according to the special circumstances of their current situation. There is a call to create a developmentally appropriate and needs-specific ESL methodology that serves two concurrent purposes: to teach the English language and to remediate for deficiencies in language development itself (Gindis, 2004, 2005). In other words, the ESL curriculum should be academic and remedial at the same time: remediation is to be intertwined with academic instruction to compensate for language-related issues of IAPI children. Its focus should be on cognitive language and specific preliteracy and literacy skills with less concentration on communicative aspects because these will be learned in the families through actual communication. Due to the remedial nature of ESL instruction, the length of the program may be longer and the intensity of the instructions may be higher than in a regular ESL program.

Based on the data presented earlier, one may conclude that language functioning of IAPI is determined by the traumatic events of their past, abrupt attrition of their first language, and the stressful situation of their new language absorbing. Suddenly, literally overnight, the use of their native language is stopped in its functions, and the children must now use another language for communication, behavior regulation, learning, and reasoning. It was not their choice; the circumstances of their new lives abruptly changed and thus discontinued exposure to one language and forced them to live in the realm of another one. Out of use, the first language is subjected to attrition, and children of preschool years and older are doomed to live through the process of losing not only a tool of socialization and adaptation (their language) but also some essential skills in behavior regulation, reasoning, and academic skills, as well as elements of their identities and self-perceptions. This is a unique psychological experience that is not fully researched and understood. For some children, this process of forgetting the first language may have a positive therapeutic effect, while for many, it is a period when their cognitive and self-regulatory weaknesses consolidate into learning disabilities and emotional dysregulation.

On average, IAPI children start learning their new language 2 to 11 years later than their peers in the neighborhood and classroom. By all means, they belong to the group of ELL students, but IAPI children differ from other participants in this group in many important areas. While adoptive parents and teachers are delighted with the speed of mastering the communicative language by the majority of IAPI children, they are equally surprised and upset by the difficulties that many IAPA children have in acquiring the cognitive/academic aspect of the English language. Such academic subjects as reading, writing, and math are heavily rooted in the cognitive/academic language, and deficiency in language mastery reflects on academic performance.

Note

1. https://www2.ed.gov/about/offices/list/ocr/ell/legal.html

References

Asimina, R., Melpomeni, S., & Alexandra, T. (2017). Language and psychosocial skills of institutionalized children in Greece. *The Open Family Studies Journal, 9*, 76–87. Retrieved from https://benthamopen.com/contents/pdf/TOFAMSJ/TOFAMSJ-9-76.pdf

Baker, C. (2001). *Foundation of bilingual education and bilingualism* (3rd ed.). Clevedon, UK: Multilingual Matters Ltd.

Bardovi-Harlig, K., & Stringer, D. (2010). Variables in second language attrition. *Studies in Second Language Acquisition, 32*, 1–45.

Benilova, S. L. (2014). *Logopedia: Systemic speech disorders in children.* Moscow: MPSI 2014, Russia (in Russian).

Bolter, N., & Cohen, N. J. (2007). Language impairment and psychiatric comorbidities. *Pediatric Clinics of North America, 54*, 525–542.

Bylund, E. S. (2009). Maturational constraints and first language attrition. In *Language learning* (Vol. 59, No. 3, pp. 687–715). Cambridge: Cambridge University Press.

Clauss, D., & Baxter, S. (1997). *Post adoption survey of Russian and Eastern European children.* Belen, NM: Rainbow House International.

Collier, V. P. (1989). How long? A synthesis of research on academic achievement in second language. *TESOL Quarterly, 23*, 509–531.

Collier, V. P., & Thomas, W. P. (1989). How quickly can immigrants become proficient in school English? *Journal of Educational Issues of Language Minority Students, 5*, 26–38.

Cummins, J. (1996). *Negotiating identities: Education for empowerment in a diverse society.* Ontario, Canada: California Association for Bilingual Education.

Cummins, J. (2000). *Language, power and pedagogy: Bilingual children in the crossfire.* Clevedon, UK: Multilingual Matters Ltd.

Dalen, M. (2001). School performance among internationally adopted children in Norway. *Adoption Quarterly, 5,* 39–58.

Desmarais, C., Roeber, B. J., Smith, M. E., & Pollak, S. D. (2012). Sentence comprehension in post-institutionalized school-age children. *Journal of Speech, Language, and Hearing Research, 55,* 45–54.

Dubrovina, I. (1991). *Psychological development of children in orphanages* ("Psichologicheskoe razvitie vospitanikov v detskom dome"). Moscow: Prosveschenie Press (in the Russian language).

Eigsti, I., Weitzman, C., Schun, J., DeMarchena, A., & Casey, B. (2011). Language and cognitive outcomes in internationally adopted children. *Development and Psychopathology, 23,* 629–646.

Elleseff, T. (2011). *What parents need to know about speech-language assessment of older internationally adopted children.* Retrieved from www.smartspeechtherapy.com/what-parents-need-to-know-about-speech-language-assessment-of-older-internationally-adopted-children/

Elleseff, T. (2013). Changing trends in international adoption: Implications for speech-language pathologists. *Perspectives on Global Issues in Communication Sciences and Related Disorders, 3,* 45–53.

Francis, N. (2005). Research findings on early first language attrition: Implications for the discussion on critical periods in language acquisition. *Language Learning, 55*(3), 491–531.

Gardner, R. C. (2010). *Motivation and second language acquisition: The socio-educational model.* New York: Peter Lang Media and Communication Ltd.

Gauthier, K., & Genesee, F. (2011). Language development in internationally adopted children: A special case of early second language learning. *Child Development, 82*(3), 887–901.

Genesee, F. (2016). Introduction. In F. Genesee & A. Delcenserie (Eds.), *Starting over: The language development in internationally adopted children* (pp. 1–16). Amsterdam: John Benjamins Publishing.

Geren, J., Snedeker, J., & Ax, L. (2005). Starting over: A preliminary study of early lexical and syntactic development in internationally adopted preschoolers. *Seminars in Speech and Language, 26,* 44–53.

Gindis, B. (1998). Navigating uncharted waters: School psychologists working with internationally adopted post-institutionalized children. *NASP Communique,* September (Part I), 27(1), 6–9 and October (Part II), 27(2), 20–23.

Gindis, B. (1999a). Language-related issues for international adoptees and adoptive families. In T. Tepper, L. Hannon, & D. Sandstrom (Eds.), *International adoption: Challenges and opportunities* (pp. 98–108). Meadow Lands, PA: PNPIC.

Gindis, B. (1999b, March). The Bilingual Verbal Ability Tests (BVAT): A breakthrough in bilingual assessment: Or is it? *NASP "Communique", 27*(6), 26–27.

Gindis, B. (2004). Language development in internationally adopted children. *China Connections, 10,* 34–37.

Gindis, B. (2005). Cognitive, language, and educational issues of children adopted from overseas orphanages. *Journal of Cognitive Education and Psychology, 4*(3), 290–315.

Glennen, S. (2002). Language development and delay in internationally adopted infants and toddlers: A review. *American Journal of Speech-Language Pathology, 11,* 333–339.

Glennen, S. (2005). New arrivals: Speech and language assessment for internationally adopted infants and toddlers within the first months home. *Seminars in Speech and Language, 26,* 10–21.

Glennen, S. (2007a). Speech and language in children adopted internationally at older ages. *Perspectives on Communication Disorders in Culturally and Linguistically Diverse Populations, 14,* 17–20.

Glennen, S. (2007b). Predicting language outcomes for internationally adopted children. *Journal of Speech, Language and Hearing Research, 50,* 529–548.

Glennen, S. (2014). A longitudinal study of language and speech in children who were internationally adopted at different ages. *Language Speech & Hearing Services in Schools, 45,* 185–203.

Glennen, S. (2015). Internationally adopted children in the early school years: Relative strengths and weaknesses in language abilities. *Language, Speech, and Hearing Services in Schools, 46,* 1–13.

Glennen, S. (2016). Speech and language clinical issues in internationally adopted children. In F. Genesee & A. Delcenserie (Eds.), *Language development in internationally adopted children: Trends in language acquisition research* (pp. 147–177). Amsterdam: John Benjamins Publishing Company.

Goodman, S. B. (2013). Internationally adopted children & language-based school difficulties. *Bank Street College of Education.* Retrieved from http://educate.bankstreet.edu/independent-studies/119

Hough, S., & Kaczmarek, L. (2011). Language and reading outcomes in young children adopted from Eastern European orphanages. *Journal of Early Intervention, 33,* 51–57.

Hyltenstam, K., Bylund, E., Abrahamsson, N., & Park, H. (2009). Dominant-language replacement. The case of international adoptees. *Bilingualism: Language and Cognition, 12*(2), 121–140.

Isurin, L. (2000). Deserted island or a child's first language forgetting. *Bilingualism: Language and Cognition, 3*(2), 151–166.

Köpke, B. (2007). Language attrition at the crossroads of brain, mind, and society. In B. Köpke, M. Schmid, M. Keizer, & S. Dostert (Eds.), *Language attrition: Theoretical perspectives* (pp. 9–37). Amsterdam: John Benjamins Publishing Company.

Kouritzin, S. (1999). *Faces of first language loss.* Mahwah, NJ: Lawrence Erlbaum Associates.

Krakow, R. A., Tao, S., & Roberts, J. (2005). Adoption age effects on English language acquisition: Infants and toddlers from China. *Seminars in Speech and Language, 26,* 33–43.

Ladage, J. S. (2009). Medical issues in international adoption and their influence on language development. *Topics in Language Disorders, 29*(1), 6–17.

Levy, B. J., McVeigh, N., Marful, A., & Anderson, M. S. (2007). Inhibiting your native language: The role of retrieval-induced forgetting during second-language acquisition. *Psychological Science, 18*(1), 29–34.

Linck, J., Judith, F., Kroll, J., & Sunderman, G. (2009). Losing access to the native language while immersed in a second language: Evidence for the role of inhibition in second-language learning. *Psychological Science, 20*(12), 1507–1515.

Mason, P., & Narad, C. (2005). International adoption: A health and developmental prospective. *Seminars in Speech and Language, 26,* 1–9.

Mayberry, R., & Lock, E. (2003). Age constraints on first versus second language acquisition: Evidence for linguistic plasticity and epigenesis. *Brain and Language, 87,* 369–384.

Meese, R. L. (2002). *Children of intercountry adoption in school.* Westport, CT: Bergen & Garvey.

Nelson, C. A. (2002). Neural development and life-long plasticity. In R. Lerner, F. Jacobs, & D. Wetlieb (Eds.), *Promoting positive child, adolescent, and family development: Handbook of program and policy interventions* (pp. 31–60). Thousand Oaks, CA: Sage Publications.

Nicoladis, E., & Grabois, H. (2002). Learning English and losing Chinese: A study of a child adopted from China. *International Journal of Bilingualism, 6*(4), 441–454.

Pallier, C., Ventureyra, V., & Yoo, H.-Y. (2004). The loss of first language phonetic perception in adopted Koreans. *Journal of Neurolinguistics, 17*(1), 79–91.

Pavlenko, A. (2005). *Emotions and multilingualism.* Cambridge: Cambridge University Press.

Pavlenko, A. (2014). *The bilingual mind and what it tells us about language and thoughts.* Cambridge: Cambridge University Press.

Pearson, C. (2001). Internationally adopted children: Issues and challenges. *The ASHA Leader, 6*(19), 4–6.

Pearson, C. (2005). Influence on the development for functional and academic language in internationally adopted children. *The Family Focus: FRUA, 6*(3), 2–6.

Pearson, C. (2008). First language attrition in internationally adopted children. *Family Focus, FRUA Journal, 14*(3), 1–14.

Pearson, C. (2010). A new home, a new culture, a new language: Issues affecting SLA in older internationally adopted children. *TEIS On-Line Journal, 24*(2). (TESOL International Association: Teacher Education Interest Section).

Pierce, L., Klein, D., Chen, J.-K., Delcenserie, A., & Genesee, F. (2014). Mapping the unconscious maintenance of a lost first language. *Proceedings of the National Academy of Sciences, 111*(48), 17314–17319.

Ponitz, C., McClelland, M., Matthews, J., & Morrison, F. (2009). A structured observation of behavioral self-regulation and its contribution to kindergarten outcomes. *Developmental Psychology, 45,* 605–619.

Qi, C., & Kaiser, A. (2004). Problem behaviors of low-income children with language delays: An observation study. *Journal of Speech, Language, and Hearing Research, 47,* 595–609.

Sakai, K. (2005). Language acquisition and brain development. *Science, 310,* 815–819.

Schmid, M. S. (2002). *First language attrition, use and maintenance: The case of German Jews in anglophone countries.* Amsterdam and Philadelphia: John Benjamins Publishing Company.

Schmid, M. S. (2004). First language attrition: The methodology revised. *International Journal of Bilingualism, 8*(3), 239–255.

Schmid, M. S. (2007). The role of L1 use for L1 attrition. In B. Köpke, M. S. Schmid, M. Keijzer, & S. Dostert (Eds.), *Language attrition: Theoretical perspectives* (pp. 135–153). Amsterdam and Philadelphia: John Benjamins Publishing Company.

Schmid, M. S. (2012). First language attrition: State of the discipline and future directions. *Linguistic Approaches to Bilingualism, 3*(1), 97–116.

Schmid, M. S., & Dusseldorp, E. (2010). Quantitative analyses in a multivariate study of language attrition: The impact of extralinguistic factors. *Second Language Research, 26*(1), 125–160.

Schmid, M. S., & Köpke, B. (Eds.). (2013). *First language attrition*. Amsterdam: John Benjamins Publishing Company.

Schmid, M. S., Köpke, B., & de Bot, K. (2012). Language attrition as a complex, non-linear development. *International Journal of Bilingualism, 17*(6), 675–682.

Schmitt, E. (2010). When boundaries are crossed: Evaluating language attrition data from two perspectives. *Bilingualism: Language and Cognition, 13*(1), 63–72.

Scott, K., Roberts, J., & Glennen, S. (2011). How well do children who are internationally adopted acquire language? A meta-analysis. *Journal of Speech, Language, & Hearing Research, 54*, 1–17.

Scott, K., Roberts, J., & Krakow, R. (2008). Oral and written language development of children adopted from China. *American Journal of Speech Language Pathology, 17*, 150–160.

Spira, E., & Fischel, J. (2005). The impact of preschool inattention, hyperactivity, and impulsivity on social and academic development: A review. *Journal of Child Psychology and Psychiatry, 46*(7), 755–773.

The St. Petersburg-USA Orphanage Research Team. (2009). The effects of early social-emotional and relationship experience on the development of young orphanage children. *Monographs of the Society for Research in Child Development, 73*(3), vii–295. Publisher: John Wiley & Sons. Contributors Crockenberg, S., Rutter, M., Bakerman-Kranenburg, M., IJzendoorn, M., & Juffer, F.

Thomas, W. P., & Collier, V. P. (1997, December). *School effectiveness for language minority students*. Washington, DC: National Clearinghouse for English Language Acquisition Resource Collection Series, No. 9 (96 pp.).

Thomas, W. P., & Collier, V. P. (2002). *A national study of school effectiveness for language minority students long-term academic achievement*. Santa Cruz, CA: Center for Research on Education, Diversity and Excellence, University of California-Santa Cruz (333 pp.).

Tumanova, T., & Filicheva, T. (2017). Russian scientific trends on specific language impairment in childhood. In F. Fernandes (Ed.), *Advances in speech-language pathology, chapter 3*. Retrieved from www.intechopen.com/books/advances-in-speech-language-pathology/russian-scientific-trends-on-specific-language-impairment-in-childhood

Van Daal, J., Verhoeven, L., & van Balkom, H. (2007). Behaviour problems in children with language impairment. *Journal of Child Psychology and Psychiatry, 48*(11), 1139–1147.

Vygotsky, L. S. (1934/1986). *Thought and language* (A. Kozulin, Newly revised and Ed.). Cambridge, MA: The MIT Press.

White, E. J., Hutka, S. A., Williams, L. J., & Moreno, S. (2013). Learning, neural plasticity and sensitive periods: Implications for language acquisition, music training and transfer across the lifespan. *Frontiers in Systems Neuroscience, 7*, 90. Retrieved from www.ncbi.nlm.nih.gov/pmc/articles/PMC3834520/

Wong-Fillmore, L. (1991). When learning a second language means losing the first. *Early Childhood Research Quarterly, 6*, 323–346.

5   Cognitive Functioning of Internationally Adopted Post-Institutionalized Children

Introduction

Cognition refers to thinking processes and skills: it is the intellectual competence that allows a human being to acquire, understand, and respond to information. Cognition, as a major psychological function, includes the ability to regulate attention, remember, process information with certain speed, solve problems, organize information, communicate, and act upon information. It has an individualized nature—people are different in their cognitive capacities. Cognitive skills develop and change over time, they can be measured, strengthened/improved, or deteriorate in certain circumstances. All these abilities work in a close, interdependent fashion with emotions and motivation to allow the person to function in his or her environment.

Cognition is a developmental psychological function in humans. Cognitive development is a synergetic result of interplay between biological qualities and environmental (social in nature) properties. In the case of IAPI children, we know very little about the first factor; as for the second factor, we are aware of the environmental characteristics of neglect, deprivation, and being overloaded with traumatic experiences. The presence of adverse conditions during gestation and after birth may have long-lasting negative effects on the developing brain. Still, there are many individual differences here.

Deficits in General Cognitive Abilities and Specific Cognitive Skills in IAPI Children

Cognitive capacities of IAPI children are rather well-researched subjects. There is a seminal meta-analysis completed by Van IJzendoorn, Luijk, and Juffer (2008), titled "IQ of Children Growing Up in Children's Homes: A Meta-Analysis on IQ Delays in Orphanages." The authors stated,

> *Children growing up in institutions showed a substantial delay in IQ compared with children reared in (foster or biological) families.*

The combined effect size in 75 studies on more than 3,800 children in 19 different countries was about three-quarters of a standard deviation. The children reared in institutions showed on average an IQ of 84; the average IQ/DQ of comparison children raised in families was 104.

(p. 341)

Such factors as the age at placement in the adoptive family, the age of the child at the time of assessment, and the "geographical factor" (the country the child had been adopted from) were associated with the extent of cognitive delays (Castle et al., 1999; MacLean, 2003; Judge, 2003; Odenstad et al., 2008; Beckett, Castle, Rutter, & Sonuga-Barke, 2010; Eigsti, Weitzman, Schun, DeMarchena, & Casey, 2011). It was found that cognitive impairments persist even after placement in a socially enriched environment, but a favorable social situation of development facilitates positive gains in overall cognitive capacity of IAPI children (Van IJzendoorn, Juffer, & Klein, 2005). Longitudinal studies of these children reported a "catchup" (although in different degrees) in global cognitive functioning (Rutter, 1998; Rutter, Kreppner, & O'Connor, 2001).

To corroborate with the earlier findings, let us consider the data collected at BGCenter from 1998 through 2013 using the Universal Nonverbal Intelligence Test (Bracken & McCallum, 1998) to measure nonverbal intelligence of newly arrived adoptees from Russia and other republics of the former Soviet Union, China, Ethiopia, and countries of Central Latin America (534 cases). The average IQ measured by the UNIT was 84, with the composite score of 88% of all cases being between 82 and 87.

Comprehensive testing of IAPI children referred to the BGCenter for academic and mental health issues after living in adoptive families for more than two years (when English became the only functional language) revealed such a range of IQ scores that any "statistical average" would be misleading. (Major IQ tests were used, such as WISC-IV and later 5th Edition, WJ-IV, Cognitive, or Stanford-Binet, 5th edition.) Two factors were notable: the country of origin (children adopted from South Korea and China showed higher IQ measurements) and the age of adoption (the younger the child, the better rate of recovery), although there were substantial individual differences. Our data fully agreed with the conclusion made by Van IJzendoorn and Juffer (2006) that, despite a measurable catchup in global cognitive functioning by IAPI children, a considerable proportion of these children continued to experience enduring deficiency in general and specific domains of cognitive functioning.

It's important to note that general cognitive potential is only one, albeit essential, marker of an IAPI child's cognitive ability to succeed in school and life. Other critical indicators were the quality of the specific cognitive processes and the effectiveness of executive functions.

A review of research literature on specific cognitive domains that are particularly affected in IAPI children is rather confusing. I attempted to assemble a ranking order of specific cognitive deficits reflected in research publications and ended up with a "laundry list" that includes executive functioning, rigidity in thinking, logical reasoning, excessive concreteness of thought, concentration and attention regulation, working memory deficits, processing speed problems, etc. (Van IJzendoorn, Juffer, & Klein, 2005; Beckett et al., 2006; Bauer, Hanson, Pierson, Davidson, & Pollak, 2009; Wilson, 2012). The common finding for the majority of publications, as formulated by Behen, Helder, Rothermel, Solomon, and Chugani (2008), was that *"a substantial proportion of international adoptees under investigation (46 percent) evidenced persistent, absolute impairment in one or more domains of neurocognitive function"* (p. 453).

At the BGCenter, based on our sample of 766 children (see Chapter 1), the most common and leading specific neurocognitive deficits found in IAPI children as a group were 1) executive dysfunction, 2) cognitive/academic language, 3) working memory, and 4) processing speed. In our research of executive function in IAPI children in the age group from 7 years through 16 years at least two years after adoption (the mean of post-adoption life was 3 years and 7 months) we used Behavior Rating Inventory of Executive Function (BRIEF, Gioia, Isquith, Guy, & Kenworthy, 2000) along with Neurocognitive Assessment Battery—CNS Vital Signs (NECOG[1]). Executive function appeared as the most pronounced cognitive deficit in IAPI children: the average Global Executive Composite (consisting of Behavior Rating Index and Meta-Cognitive Index) standard score of 72 was at or below the third percentile in comparison to their age peers in the standardization sample.

It is hardly possible to pinpoint the specific cause(s) of a particular cognitive deficit in IAPI children: every case is always a result of an early biological vulnerability combined with an adverse developmental experience coalesced in various proportions. We still do not know a precise path through which early caregiving shapes the executive functions, but the research had already pointed at the broad impact of early caregiving on the development of neural systems involved in executive function, particularly on prefrontal circuitry (Camelia et al., 2012).

Cognitive Profile of IAPI Children With FASD

In the context of cognitive profiling, IAPI children with fetal alcohol syndrome disorder (FASD), were specifically studied in our clinic. In general, our findings are basically congruent with the conclusion of the meta-analysis conducted by Kodituwakku (2009) who found that

> *children with FASD show diminished intellectual functioning, with average IQ scores falling within the borderline to low average ranges.*

Slow information processing and disturbances of attention have been observed from infancy through adulthood in individuals with FASD. Clinical and experimental reports on individuals with FASD have documented marked deficits in executive functioning, particularly in tasks that involve holding and manipulating information in working memory. Studies examining specific domains of cognitive functioning such as language, visual perception, memory and learning, social functioning, and number processing in individuals with FASD have revealed performance decrements associated with increased task complexity. The above findings converge on the conclusion that children with FASD have a generalized deficit in the processing and integration of information.

(p. 218)

Still, a cognitive profile of IAPI children afflicted by FASD has a specificity not found in their peers with the same condition in the general population.

The overall number of subjects in our research study was 63: 27 girls (43%) and 36 boys (57%) adopted from Russia (72%), Ukraine, Kazakhstan, Moldova, Estonia, and Latvia. The ages ranged from 5 years to 16 years with the median of adoption age (time with adoptive families) at 4 years and 8 months. Fifteen out of 63 cases were longitudinal: from two to three consecutive assessments within the 3 to 9 years. General cognitive abilities were measured using the WISC-IV and WISC-5 (in six cases through UNIT). Specific cognitive processes, such as speed of processing and working memory, measured by means of a "cross-battery approach" (McGrew, Ortiz, & Flanagan, 2001) using relevant subtests from UNIT, NEPSY-II, WJ-IV, Cognitive, and Neurocognitive Assessment Battery—CNS Vital Signs (NECOG-VS). Executive functions were assessed through BRIEF and selected tests from NEPSY-II and NECOG-VS.

In our sample, as presented in the graph that follows, general cognitive ability was in the range of 76 to 92, with an average score of 82 (Low Average to Borderline range). Composite adaptive behavior standard scores fell in the range of 67 to 80, with an average score of 75 (Borderline range). Total achievement standard scores were in the 82 to 96 range, with an average score of 91 (Average to Low Average range).

Processing speed measurements revealed a rather wide range (77 to 109), with the arithmetical average of 93 being somewhat unrepresentative. The majority of examinees performed close to their respective age norms (mostly in the Low Average to Average range) in simple grapho-motor tasks, like Visual Matching (WJ-IV, Cognitive) or Coding (WISC-IV and WISC-5). However, for more cognitively challenging assignments that depended on the application of speedy and accurate high-order reasoning in a systematic goal-directed behavior, the outcome was far below average for age norms. Working memory and processing speed fell within a broad range of standard scores from 72 to 99, with an average of 85. Standard scores in executive functions, on the other hand, were in the rather narrow range of 60 to 74, with an average of 67.

As seen in Table 5.1, the academic achievements are higher than corresponding cognitive scores: in our sample, we consistently observed the reverse cognition-achievement discrepancy. It is likely that remedial efforts by the parents and teachers payoff: the students with limitations in their cognitive capacity perform higher than expected on academic tasks.

As seen in Table 5.2, the executive functions constitute a major cognitive deficit in the IAPI children affected by FASD. On the other hand, the processing speed in simple visual tasks appears to be their relative strength, which is important for the future occupational training.

Table 5.1 Basic Psychological Functions IAPI Children With FASD

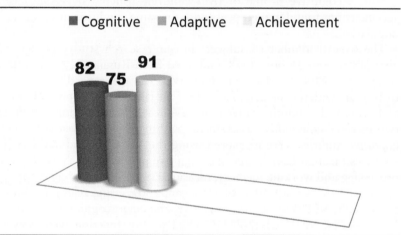

Table 5.2 Specific Psychological Functions IAPI Children With FASD

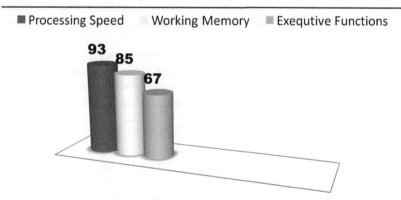

The research literature identifies slow processing speed (Burden, Jacobson, & Jacobson, 2005), limited attention (McGee, Schonfeld, Roebuck-Spencer, Riley, & Mattson, 2008), restricted working memory (Rasmussen, 2005), and difficulties with high-order reasoning as typical for children with FASD (Matson, Crocker, & Nguyen, 2011). Our data only partially confirms these findings.

We found that the composite cognitive "profile" of IAPI children in our cohort, obtained by major standardized test batteries, is diverse, complex, and subject to individual differences. What was common for practically all IAPI children in our sample is that in assignments where self-regulation of cognitive processes required goal-directed systematic performance, their scores lowered almost uniformly. Thus, our subjects demonstrated distinct difficulties in regulating attention and sustaining attention in a goal-directed activity. It appears that limitations in cognitive functioning could be found mostly in a limited ability to self-regulate cognitive processes.

Practically all subjects in our sample had difficulties with high-order (abstract) reasoning. In early elementary school, this is not as obvious, and they can make it through those years without noticeable differences. After the age of 10–11, however, both cognitive tests and academic assignments rely more heavily on abstract thinking, and subjects in our sample begin to fall behind the norms designed for their nonhandicapped peers.

While IAPI children with FASD present a range of cognitive abilities, the majority fall in the Low Average to Borderline category. As academic and psychological tests become more complex and abstract in nature, those in the Low Average range struggle and slip into the Borderline range of general cognitive ability. This may produce an impression of "deterioration," but in fact, it is a specific and typical dynamic of cognitive/academic functioning for individuals with FASD: the pace of their cognitive development does not conform to societal expectations for certain age groups (Gindis, 2014).

Cumulative Cognitive Deficit as a Specific Feature of the Cognitive Profile of IAPI Children

Adoptive parents and teachers of school-age international adoptees often express their concerns and frustrations over the slower than expected academic progress of these children in school. After an initial phase of seemingly fast new language acquisition and adjustment to their new homes and schools, many international adoptees have significant difficulty in their academic work, which, in turn, leads to behavioral and emotional problems. Their learning difficulties may persist and worsen long past the time when their academic problems could be attributed to new language learning and adjustment issues. Moreover, as international adoptees progress through the developmental stages and school grades, many of them seem to fall farther and farther behind age norms in their performance on academic tasks and intelligence tests. In some international adoptees, the overall pace of cognitive and language development and academic performance is too slow or inconsistent and fails to match comprehensive and relentless efforts of their adoptive parents and professionals in different fields (Clauss & Baxter, 1997; Gindis, 1998, 2006; Connor & Rutter, 1999; Price, 2000; Dole, 2005; Meese, 2002, 2005; Welsh & Viana, 2012).

Definition and Structure of Cumulative Cognitive Deficit

One of the compelling explanations of this phenomenon is that these children experience what is known as "cumulative cognitive deficit" (CCD), a term coined by psychologist Martin Deutsch in the 1960s (Jachuck & Mohanty, 1974; Cox, 1983). CCD is a psychological construct referring to a downward trend in the measured intelligence and scholastic achievement of culturally/socially disadvantaged children relative to age-appropriate societal norms and expectations. The evidence of CCD existence comes from a variety of sources (Jensen, 1974, 1977; Kamin, 1978; Saco-Pollitt, Pollitt, & Greenfield, 1985), and the theory behind CCD is that "*children who are deprived of enriching cognitive experiences during their early years are less able to profit from environmental situations because of a mismatch between their cognitive schemata and the requirements of the new advanced learning situation*" (Sattler, 1992, pp. 575–576).

In the context of post-adoption cognitive functioning of IAPI children, the publication of Wohlwill (1980) was noteworthy. The author stated that the major critical factor in the formation of CCD is the continuation of the deprived environmental conditions to which the children are exposed. He suggested that merely a change of environment (e. g.: placement of a child afflicted with CCD in a cognitively more advantageous environment) may ameliorate the deficit. He hypothesized that in a more stimulating environment, the cognitive deficit will decrease by itself, resulting in an age-appropriate cognitive/academic performance. Only ten years after Wohlwill's prediction, a massive "natural experiment" (international adoption) began and has revealed that a mere improvement of environment does not eliminate CCD: a significant group among IAPI children continues to demonstrate full-blown CCD after years living in what Wohlwill called an "advantageous environment."

An analysis of empirical research on CCD in research publications (Haywood, 1987; Mackner, Starr, & Black, 1997; Castle et al., 1999; O'Connor, Rutter, Beckett, Keaveney, & Kreppner, 2000; Gindis, 2006; Nelson et al., 2007) revealed the following major characteristics of this phenomenon:

- A lack of age-appropriate cognitive skills leading to progressive cognitive/behavioral incompetence. Specifically, limited or nonexistent meta-cognitive skills, such as monitoring one's own thinking or learning how to study by mastering learning strategies and methods.

- Poor organization of knowledge base resulting in ineffective learning, constant forgetting of learned material, and inability to transfer knowledge and skills from one situation to another.
- Cognitive/academic language deficiency often existing concurrently with the fully functional social "everyday" language.
- Chronic mismatch between the student's learning aptitude and his or her learning environment, level of instructions, and the manner of the teacher's presentation and instruction.

The core root of CCD in IAPI children constitutes severe educational and cultural deprivation—a lack of direct and mediated learning in early childhood—combined with a host of trauma-producing factors.

Young children learn in two major ways: directly (through observing, experimenting, experiencing, and imitating) and indirectly (through adults who mediate knowledge for children by selecting and modifying input from the outside world and directing children's responses). Through direct and mediated learning, major cognitive skills and processes are formed and put in action. Deprived of such experiences, children are indeed disadvantaged and may have problems moving to more advanced levels of learning. When a child misses certain stages of normal cognitive development and never learns generic concepts necessary for successful schooling, the educational matter this child is taught simply does not have any structural support upon which to be understood, remembered, and used. No wonder: all high-order cognitive abilities (abstract thinking/concept formation, analysis/synthesis, perceptual organization, sequential/simultaneous processing, symbolic mediation, etc.) are developmentally hierarchical. The appearance of more complex cognitive structures rests upon the prior emergence of simpler cognitive components; e.g., the ability to compare appears prior to classifying, classifying prior to seriating, and so on (Bruner, 1966). The psychological roots of CCD are developed in the absence of a viable foundation for productive development of more complex cognitive skills and processes. For example, elementary cognitive skills like patterning or sequencing, normally are formed between the ages 3 to 5 in a typically developing child through direct experience and mediated learning (Rittle-Johnson, Fyfe, McLean, & McEldoon, 2013). As our clinical experience revealed, the same patterning/sequencing understanding is often absent in a 7- or 8-year-old former orphanage resident (Gindis & Karpov, 2000). However, more complex math and reading skills rest on these basic cognitive notions, so without rebuilding the base, no successful remediation is possible. Unfortunately, traditional remediation in schools simply assumes the presence of an appropriate base and tries to build compensatory structures upon it.

CCD in the population at large is traditionally associated with children from poor and uneducated families. Most internationally adopted children now live in middle-class families with well-educated parents. Probably for the first time in the history of CCD, families are not ongoing contributing factors to this phenomenon; on the contrary, they may be considered as a powerful curative factor for CCD remediation. Due to adoptive parents' sensitivity to and awareness of possible learning problems in international adoptees and because of higher parental expectations in this respect, symptoms of CCD are reported and treated earlier by professionals in such situations (Van IJzendoorn & Juffer, 2006; Gindis, 1998, 2006; Welsh, Andres, Viana, Petrill, & Mathias, 2007).

As mentioned earlier, traditionally, the causes of CCD have been attributed mostly (if not exclusively) to a "culture of poverty"—that is, to ongoing cultural/educational deprivation. In contrast to this single cause approach, the determinants of CCD in international adoptees may be associated with a combination of factors, such as developmental trauma disorder, neurological weakness, educational/cultural neglect and deprivation in early childhood, abrupt first-language attrition, inappropriate learning environment (e.g., a lack of remedial education), etc. Consequently, the remedial efforts should be multifaceted.

The study of CCD in IAPI children gives us an opportunity to see this phenomenon from a new angle, when the social situation of their development has been changed for the best practically overnight, but the nature and dynamics of CCD have persisted due to inner, deeply ingrained causes. The CCD in IAPI children may be different in certain aspects from what we know about CCD in the population at large, and this uniqueness must be recognized and addressed in our remedial efforts. Let us consider a clinical case of an internationally adopted child who experiences the CCD.

Case Study: Alyona—An Older IAPI Child With CCD

Alyona was adopted at the age of 8, having completed the first grade in her native Russia. She had been brought to an orphanage at birth. Although Alyona was below the fifth percentile for her age in height and weight, she was described as a "practically healthy" child at the time of her adoption. According to her medical record, in her early childhood, Alyona suffered from anemia (iron deficiency), rickets (vitamin D deficiency), moderate malnutrition (underweight), and delays in gross-motor development. Her medical record also carried a diagnosis of "delays in psychological and language development," which was almost a standard feature for children who had come from Russian orphanages (Gindis, 1998).

Alyona was examined at the BGCenter within a month of her arrival in the USA in order to verify this diagnosis and recommend the appropriate academic placement for her. She was tested by a licensed psychologist with native fluency and proper certification in the Russian language. The first assessment was performed mostly with nonverbal tests and with verbal testing in the child's native language. The examiner made a note that no evidence of neurological impairment was found in Alyona during a brief examination by a developmental neurologist prior to her psychoeducational assessment.

At the time of her initial psychological evaluation, Alyona was a monolingual (Russian only) child. It was impossible in any meaningful way to quantify the intellectual abilities of this non-English-speaking child with an atypical background through standardized testing. Alyona's academic skills were measured informally against the Russian curriculum (preschool to grade 1) in language, math, and general knowledge. She was found to have unevenly developed and rather delayed literacy skills, being an "emerging reader" at best. Her social-adaptive behavior estimated in terms of skills in daily living, self-help, socialization, and gross/fine motor skills appeared age-appropriate. Her intelligence was tested with the Universal Nonverbal Intelligence Test (UNIT), and her verbal cognitive functioning was examined through several classical Piagetian and Vygotskian tasks (presented orally in Russian) on hierarchical classification, comprehension of sequential events, understanding of "double-meaning" expressions, generalization, and abstraction (see this procedure in Gindis & Karpov, 2000). Alyona's performance, although inconsistent, was within the Average to Low Average range. Nevertheless, evidences of notable cognitive limitations were found in her verbal comprehension and such cognitive operations as associations, categorization, classification, or discrimination. Her particular weakness was in sequential skills: it was difficult for her to recall auditory and visual information in proper sequence and detail, and to apply cognitive strategies that require step-by-step procedures. Like a much younger child, Alyona needed constant visual references to support her understanding or reasoning. Although her communicative fluency in her native language was close to her age expectations, her ability to use language as a tool for her own mental operations was limited, immature, and ineffective. At that time, Alyona's relative weakness in cognitive skills was attributed to her background of deprivation, and her cognitive potential was estimated as being close to age-expected norms. In spite of the obvious mismatch between Alyona's level of functioning and the demands of her new school setting (one of the best in New York state), she was placed, according to her age, in a regular third grade class with ESL services.

Aloyna's next testing took place two years later, this time requested by the school district due to her "slow progress" in academic subjects. Alyona again was virtually a monolingual child, this time in the English language. She was tested by the same bilingual (Russian/English) psychologist as during her initial screening. It was confirmed that Alyona had completely lost her native language, not only in the expressive mode but also in the receptive one, to say nothing of her literacy skills—a rather typical case for IAPI children of her age and circumstances (Gindis, 2008). Although her communicative fluency in English seemed to be at least functional, her cognitive/academic English was very limited: as measured by the Woodcock-Muñoz Language Survey—Revised Normative Update (WMLS-R NU, 2010), her standard score was 72 and grade equivalent was below the first grade. Her academic level in reading, writing, and math was three to four grades below her current academic placement (fifth grade). It was judged by the examiner that, because of practically full attrition of Alyona's first language, English was the only language she had at the time of that assessment. Her level of acculturation after more than two years of life in her adoptive middle-class family was sufficient enough to offer her cognitive testing using the Wechsler Intelligence Scale for Children, Fourth Edition (WISC-IV). Standardized testing using WISC-IV showed a Low Average to Borderline level of intellectual functioning. An analysis of her performance revealed many cognitive deficiencies, particularly with processing speed, working memory, and spatial/temporal sequencing. She demonstrated poor comprehension of notion/concept meaning, and limited ability to recall or memorize any abstract material. Her test-taking behavior was quite immature: she engaged in impulsive and disorganized "exploratory" actions, mostly through "trial-and-error" attempts. Her attention, motivation, and ability to tolerate frustration in cognitive activities were less sustained than two years earlier. It was obvious that Alyona had not taken full advantage of her new environment: her cognitive functioning was progressing too slowly in comparison with the changing demands of her educational setting. A comprehensive remedial program was recommended—that included special education placement, specific remedial methodologies for reading and math, supportive services, language therapy, and classroom accommodations—but was rejected by the school on the grounds of "not qualifying for Individual Educational Plan."

A year later, mostly due to Alyona's escalating behavior problems (anger, refusal to participate in classroom activities, failure to submit homework, etc.) her adoptive parents initiated a new comprehensive psychoeducational evaluation. Alyona's progress was discussed again vis-à-vis the requirements of her current grade curriculum. She made only a few gains in her academic achievement, and her deficit in cognitive functioning continued to increase. An examination completed by a school psychologist using the Stanford-Binet Intelligence Test (5th Edition) revealed estimated intelligence in the Borderline to Mentally Deficient range, a significant decline from her previous assessments. Alyona's teachers reported weak language skills in reading and writing activities, poor comprehension of abstract notions and concepts, incompetence in many age-appropriate mental activities, constant "tiredness," "daydreaming," and "boredom" in class, which were in sharp contrast to her keen interest and energy in social situations and sports activities. There was an obvious disparity between Alyona's current instructional setting and her ability to benefit from it. It appeared as if she was "racing against time," being unable to catchup with age-level academic standards and respond adequately to the intensity of remedial efforts. Because of the discrepancy between steadily rising academic requirements and relatively slow cognitive and language growth, her overall cognitive/academic trend seemed to be a "downward" one. There was an obvious disparity between her current instructional setting and her ability to benefit from it. This time, the educational classification "learning disabled" was assigned and the remedial work was spelled out in Alyona's Individual Educational Plan. However, valuable time had been lost.

The Contributing Factors for CCD in IAPI Children

Alyona's case illustrates the essential qualities of CCD in international adoptees: it is a complex phenomenon, a combination of the internal factors (the consequences of DTD, abrupt language attrition, combination of innate and socially induced cognitive limitations, lack of motivation) and the external circumstances (inadequate teaching methods and learning environment). To complicate the picture further, due to its "summative" nature, CCD can go undetected in the early stages of the child's educational journey: it takes time for the cognitive deficit to consolidate and become "cumulative." In addition, there are at least four contributing factors, listed next, that make CCD in IAPI children really unique and even more challenging for remediation.

Neurological Weaknesses

Neurological weaknesses of IAPI children, described in the previous chapters, constitute the biological background of their cognitive limitations and are observable in many "soft" neurological signs, inability to concentrate and be attentive, and fatigue and nervous tension during mental efforts. Certain medical disorders, such as anxiety, depression, PTSD, ADHD, mood dysregulation, or bipolar disorder may reinforce CCD.

Emotional/Motivational Factors

Learning always includes the emotional and motivational components that mediate cognitive functioning. This factor was practically ignored in the literature on CCD, with the exception of an article published by C. H. Haywood (1987), where the author wrote, "*Constant failure in cognitive/ academic activities . . . feeds upon itself in a negative spiraling fashion which results in low self-esteem and/or lack of interest in and constant frustration associated with cognitive efforts*" (p. 198).

Indeed, at times, it is difficult to differentiate between primary (is it mostly cognitive?) and secondary (is it mostly emotional?) disabilities in an internationally adopted child referred for "learning" problems. It appears likely that emotional/behavioral and cognitive difficulties are tightly intertwined and constitute a very important characteristic of CCD in post-institutionalized children.

Abrupt First-Language Attrition and Failure to Transfer Cognitive Skills From One Language to the Other

Still another contributing factor to the CCD in IAPI children is the abrupt first-language attrition and the specificity of new language learning in international adoptees. This theme was considered in Chapter 4 of this book. In brief, language is a medium through which cognitive skills and knowledge are formed, present, and further developed. Abrupt first-language attrition prevents the successful "transfer" of cognitive skills from the first language to the new one (Gindis, 2008). Also, their tempo of losing native language and acquiring the new one does not dovetail: clinical data indicates that cognitive difficulties may be exacerbated with a cumulative effect during the time when the first language is lost for all practical purposes with the second language barely functional communicatively and not in existence cognitively (Schaerlaekens, 1998; Gindis, 1998; Eigsti et al., 2011; Spratt et al., 2012). The overall length of this period depends on the children's age and a host of individual differences, but for many IAPI children, this is the time when their cognitive weaknesses are consolidated into a CCD.

Cross-Cultural Component of CCD in Older IAPI Children

Among so-called older international adoptees who are adopted at school-age (currently about one-quarter of adopted children), there is a certain cross-cultural component of CCD. The value of cognitive activity, intrinsic motivation in cognitive operations, learning behavior in general, and attitude toward teaching authority may be influenced by the initial (native) base culture (see more on this topic in Haywood, 2005). On the other hand, we have to realize that CCD in international adoptees is diagnosed on the basis of US middle-class norms and expectations. The cultural differences of IAPI school-age children can contribute to cognitive functioning, at least during the initial adjustment period.

At what age can CCD be diagnosed? In fact, CCD needs time to become "cumulative"; therefore, the earliest time is the beginning of elementary school—second or third grade. Full-blown CCD, however, is normally observed in third to fifth grade—ages 8–12. The likelihood of CCD in IAPI children adopted at school-age is high, but there is no statistical data on this matter. Remedial education is the most effective way to address CCD in IAPI children. An appropriate academic placement and remediation are needed to prevent further deterioration in learning capacity and motivation to learn.

Note

1. www.cnsvs.com/

References

Bauer, P. M., Hanson, J. L., Pierson, R. K., Davidson, R. J., & Pollak, S. D. (2009). Cerebellar volume and cognitive functioning in children who experienced early deprivation. *Biological Psychiatry*, 66, 1100–1106.

Beckett, C., Castle, J., Rutter, M., & Sonuga-Barke, E. J. (2010). Institutional deprivation, specific cognitive functions, and scholastic achievement: English and Romanian Adoptee (ERA) study findings. *Monographs of the Society for Research in Child Development*, 75, 125–142.

Beckett, C., Maughan, B., Rutter, M., Castle, J., Colvert, F., & Groothues, C. (2006). Do the effects of early severe deprivation on cognition persist into early adolescence? Findings from the English and Romanian Adoptees Study. *Child Development*, 77, 696–711.

Behen, M. E., Helder, E., Rothermel, R., Solomon, K., & Chugani, H. T. (2008). Incidence of specific absolute neurocognitive impairment in globally intact children with histories of early severe deprivation. *Child Neuropsychology*, 14, 453–469.

Bracken, B. A., & McCallum, R. S. (1998). *Universal nonverbal intelligence test*. Itasca, IL: Riverside Publishing.

Bruner, J. (1966). *Toward a theory of instruction*. Cambridge, MA: Harvard University Press.

Burden, M. J., Jacobson, S. W., & Jacobson, J. L. (2005). Relation of prenatal alcohol exposure to cognitive processing speed and efficiency in childhood. *Alcoholism: Clinical and Experimental Research*, 29(8), 1473–1483.

Camelia, E., Hostinar, C., Stellern, S., Schaefer, C., Carlson, S., Megan, R., & Gunnar, M. (2012). Associations between early life adversity and executive function in children adopted internationally. *Proceedings of the National Academy of Sciences*, 109(2), 7208–17212.

Castle, J., Groothues, C., Bredenkamp, D., Beckett, C., O'Connor, T., & Rutter, M. (1999). Effects of qualities of early institutional care on cognitive attainment. *American Journal of Orthopsychiatry*, 69(4), 424–437.

Clauss, D., & Baxter, S. (1997). *Post adoption survey of Russian and Eastern European children*. Belen, NM: Rainbow House International.

Connor, T., & Rutter, M. (1999). Effects of qualities of early institutional care on cognitive attainment. *American Journal of Orthopsychiatry*, 69(4), 424–437.

Cox, T. (1983). Cumulative deficit in culturally disadvantaged children. *British Journal of Educational Psychology*, 53(3), 317–326.

Dole, K. N. (2005). Education and internationally adopted children: Working collaboratively with schools. *Pediatric Clinics of North America*, 52, 1445–1461.

Eigsti, I., Weitzman, C., Schun, J., DeMarchena, A., & Casey, B. (2011). Language and cognitive outcomes in internationally adopted children. *Development and Psychopathology*, 23, 629–646.

Gindis, B. (1998). Navigating uncharted waters: School psychologists working with internationally adopted post-institutionalized children. *NASP Communiqué*, Part I: 27(1), 6–9; Part II: 27(2), 20–23.

Gindis, B. (2006). Cognitive, language, and educational issues of children adopted from overseas orphanages. *Journal of Cognitive Education and Psychology, 4*(3), 290–315.

Gindis, B. (2008). Abrupt native language loss in international adoptees. *ADVANCE for Speech-Language Pathologists and Audiologists, 18,* 5–13.

Gindis, B. (2014). Psychological characteristics of internationally adopted post-institutionalized children with Fetal Alcohol Spectrum Disorders. *The International Journal of Alcohol and Drug Research, 3*(1), 35–42.

Gindis, B., & Karpov, Y. (2000). Dynamic assessment of the level of internalization of elementary school children's problem-solving activity. In C. Lidz & J. Elliott (Eds.), *Dynamic assessment: Prevailing models and applications* (pp. 133–154). Oxford, UK: Elsevier Science.

Gioia, G., Isquith, P., Guy, S., & Kenworthy, L. (2000). Behavior rating inventory of executive function. *Child Neuropsychology, 6*(3), 235–238.

Haywood, H. C. (1987). The mental age deficit: Explanation and treatment. *Upsala Journal of Medical Science, 44,* 191–203.

Haywood, H. C. (2005). Transculturality and cognitive development: Some observations and some questions. *Journal of Cognitive Education and Psychology, 4*(3), 273–289.

Jachuck, K., & Mohanty, A. K. (1974). Low socio-economic status and progressive retardation in cognitive skills: A test of cumulative deficit hypothesis. *Journal of Mental Retardation, 7*(1), 36–45.

Jensen, A. R. (1974). Cumulative deficit: A testable hypothesis? *Developmental Psychology, 10,* 996–1019.

Jensen, A. R. (1977). Cumulative deficit in IQ of blacks in the rural South. *Developmental Psychology, 13,* 184–191.

Judge, S. (2003). Developmental recovery and deficit in children adopted from Eastern European Orphanages. *Child Psychiatry and Human Development, 34,* 49–62.

Kamin, L. J. (1978). A positive reinterpretation of apparent "cumulative deficit". *Developmental Psychology, 14,* 195–196.

Kodituwakku, P. (2009). Neurocognitive profile in children with fetal alcohol spectrum disorders. *Developmental Disability Research Review, 15*(3), 218–224.

Mackner, L. M., Starr, R. H., & Black, M. (1997). The cumulative effect of neglect and failure to thrive on cognitive functioning. *Child Abuse & Neglect, 21*(7), 691–700.

MacLean, K. (2003). The impact of institutionalization on child development. *Development and Psychopathology, 15,* 853–884.

Matson, S., Crocker, N., & Nguyen, T. (2011). Fetal alcohol spectrum disorders: Neuropsychological and behavioral features. *Neuropsychology Review, 21*(2), 81–101.

McGee, C., Schonfeld, A., Roebuck-Spencer, T., Riley, E., & Mattson, S. (2008). Children with heavy prenatal alcohol exposure demonstrate deficits on multiple measures of concept formation. *Alcoholism: Clinical and Experimental Research, 32*(8), 1388–1397.

McGrew, K., Ortiz, S., & Flanagan, D. (2001). *Essentials of cross-battery assessment.* New York: Wiley & Sons.

Meese, R. L. (2002). *Children of intercountry adoptions in school: A primer for parents and professionals*. Westport, CT: Bergin & Garvey.

Meese, R. L. (2005). A few new children: Post-institutional children of intercounty adoption. *The Journal of Special Education, 39*(3), 157–167.

Nelson, C. A., Zeanah, C. H., Fox, N. A., Marshall, P. J., Smyke, A., & Guthrie, D. (2007). Cognitive recovery in socially deprived young children: The Bucharest Early Intervention Project. *Science, 318*, 1937–1940.

O'Connor, T. G., Rutter, M., Beckett, C., Keaveney, L., & Kreppner, J. M. (2000). The effects of global severe privation on cognitive competence: Extension and longitudinal follow-up: English & Romanian adoptees study team. *Child Development, 71*, 376–390.

Odenstad, A., Hjern, A., Lindblad, E., Rasmussen, E., Vinnerljung, B., & Dalen, M. (2008). Does age at adoption and geographic origin matter? A national cohort study of cognitive test performance in adult inter-country adoptees. *Psychological Medicine, 38*, 1803–1814.

Price, P. (2000). FRUA's health and development survey. *The Family Focus, 6*(3), 1–3.

Rasmussen, C. (2005). Executive and working memory in fetal alcohol spectrum disorder. *Alcohol Clinical Experimental Research, 29*(8), 1359–1367.

Rittle-Johnson, E., Fyfe, E., McLean, L., & McEldoon, K. (2013). Emerging understanding of patterning in 4-year-olds. *Journal of Cognition and Development, 14*(3), 375–395.

Rutter, M. L. (1998). Developmental catch-up, and deficit, following adoption after severe global early privation. *Journal of Child Psychology & Psychiatry, 39*, 465–476.

Rutter, M. L., Kreppner, J. M., & O'Connor, T. J. (2001). Specificity and heterogeneity in children's responses to profound institutional privation. *British Journal of Psychiatry, 179*, 97–103.

Saco-Pollitt, C., Pollitt, E., & Greenfield, D. (1985). The cumulative deficit hypothesis in the light of cross-cultural evidence. *International Journal of Behavioral Development, 8*(1), 75–97.

Sattler, J. M. (1992). *Assessment of children* (Revised and updated 3rd ed.). San Diego: Jerome M. Sattler, Publisher.

Schaerlaekens, A. (1998). Language adjustment in international adoptions: An exploratory study. *Journal of Multilingual and Multicultural Development, 9*(3), 247–266.

Spratt, E., Friedenberg, S., LaRosa, A., Bellis, M., Macias, M., Summer, A., . . . Brady, K. (2012). The effects of early neglect on cognitive, language, and behavioral functioning in childhood. *Scientific Research: Psychology, 3*(2), 175–182.

Van IJzendoorn, M. H., & Juffer, E. (2006). The Emanuel Miller memorial lecture 2006: Adoption as intervention. Meta-analytic evidence for massive catch-up and plasticity in physical, socio-emotional, and cognitive development. *Journal of Child Psychology and Psychiatry, 47*, 1228–1245.

Van IJzendoorn, M. H., Juffer, E., & Klein, P. (2005). Adoption and cognitive development: A meta-analytic comparison of adopted and nonadopted children's IQ and school performance. *Psychological Bulletin, 13*, 301–316.

Van Ijzendoorn, M. H., Luijk, M., & Juffer, F. (2008). IQ of children growing up in children's homes: A meta-analysis on IQ delays in orphanages. *Merrill-Palmer Quarterly, 54*(3), 341–366.

Welsh, J., Andres, G., Viana, A., Petrill, S., & Mathias, M. (2007). Interventions for internationally adopted children and families: A review of the literature. *Child and Adolescent Social Work Journal, 24.*

Welsh, J., & Viana, A. (2012). Developmental outcomes of internationally adopted children. *Adoption Quarterly, 15*(4), 241–264.

Wilson, S. (2012). Cognitive development. In D. Hwa-Froelich (Ed.), *Supporting development in internationally adopted children*. Baltimore, MD: Paul H. Brookers Publishing.

Wohlwill, J. H. (1980). Cognitive development in childhood. In O. G. Brim, Jr. & J. Kagan (Eds.), *Constancy and change in human development*. Cambridge, MA: Harvard University Press.

6 Social/Emotional and Behavioral Functioning of Internationally Adopted Post-Institutionalized Children

Introduction

According to a massive volume of research literature, IAPI children have more behavioral issues and social/emotional difficulties than their non-adopted peers. Thus Keys, Sharma, Elkins, Iacono, and McGue (2008) concluded, "*Being internationally adopted approximately doubled the odds of having contact with a mental health professional*" (p. 419). Indeed, IAPI children are disproportionally presented in admission entries to mental health facilities (Juffer & van IJzendoorn, 2005). There are several meta-analytical studies that have indicated that IAPI children have

- significantly higher rates of *internalizing problems*, such as depression and anxiety (Juffer & van IJzendoorn, 2005; Tarullo, Bruce, & Gunnar, 2007; Hostinar, Stellern, Schaefer, & Gunnar, 2012);
- higher rates of social problems with peers and adults than children raised by their biological families (Gunnar & van Dulmen, 2007; Stevens, Sonuga-Barke, Kreppner, Beckett, & Castle, 2007)
- increased rates of behavioral problems from middle childhood to adolescence (Colvert et al., 2008; Tieman, van der Ende, and Verhulst (2005); and
- behavioral problems as the greatest challenge among children who were older (after the age of 5) at the time of their adoption, who were exposed to a more prolonged institutional deprivation, or who have special needs (Wright & Flynn, 2006; Merz & McCall, 2010).

Post-institutionalized children have been reported to display a variety of atypical behaviors, including stereotyped self-stimulation and "autistic-like" patterns of behavior, swinging between passivity and aggressiveness, distractibility, inability to form deep and genuine attachments, indiscriminate friendliness, and difficulty establishing appropriate peer relationships. (Hoksbergen, Rijk, van Dijkum, & ter Laak, 2004; Juffer & van IJzendoorn, 2005; Rutter et al., 2007; Bruce, Tarullo, & Gunnar, 2009).

Behavioral problems can be grouped as short term (temporary) and long term (consistent and difficult to overcome). Certain problems apparent at the time of adoption tend to be temporary, including eating problems (e.g., refusal of solid foods, overeating) or self-stimulating behaviors. On the other hand, certain problems may increase over the years following adoption, especially the internalized behavior problems related to social and peer relations, and regulating emotions, anger, and aggression (Kreppner, O'Connor, & Rutter, 2001; Merz & McCall, 2010).

N. Zill (2017) examined a longitudinal study of 19,000 students that was conducted by the National Center for Education Statistics beginning in 1998. He found that, as measured by their teachers, young adopted children were more likely to get angry easily and to fight with other students than their peers from biological families. If a 50% score represented an average level of this type of "problem behavior," adopted kindergarteners were higher than average at 64%, while children with two biological parents were at 44%. Children in single-parent, step, and foster families all had fewer behavioral issues than adopted kindergarteners. A similar pattern (63% versus 43%) emerged for adopted and biological first graders. Teachers also noted that adopted children were less likely to pay attention in class, were less eager to learn new things, and didn't persist as needed long on challenging tasks (Zill, 2017).

What is worth noting is that the strongest positive associations between age at adoption and social problems were found during adolescence rather than when the same children were assessed at younger ages. Thus older-adopted IAPI adolescents often have immature self-regulatory skills that negatively affect successful transitions to young adulthood. Furthermore, older-adopted IAPI adolescents are often found impaired in their social skills, which may put them at a disadvantage during a developmental period that emphasizes peer interactions (Gleitman & Savaya, 2011).

Review of the research literature and clinical experience suggest that the major factor influencing IAPI child's behavior and social/emotional functioning is a combined effect of the pre-adoption profound childhood trauma and the post-adoption traumatic experience in the new family and at school.

Pre-Adoptive Childhood Trauma and Later Behavioral Difficulties

A significant number of studies indicate that adverse childhood experience before adoption, such as neglect, deprivation, and institutionalization, can have a detrimental effect on the behavioral adjustment of adoptees, particularly on those adopted after 3 to 5 years of age (Nemeroff, 2004; Merz & McCall, 2010; Ji, Brooks, Barth, & Kim, 2010; Hawk & McCall, 2011; Grotevant & McDermott, 2014). The psychological impact of early trauma on children's behavior (fully applicable to international adoptees) was explained by Cozolino (2014, p. 136) this way:

> *The roots of behavior issues are in the early sensory-motor (bodily) and emotional remembrances of infants and toddlers. The collective work of the amygdala, thalamus, cerebellum, and orbital medial prefrontal structures organizes and retains primitive vestibular-sensory-emotional memories of early caretaking, rendering them of permanent psychological significance. These early implicit memories come to serve as the emotional background against which the subsequent psychological development takes place.*

As the brain matures, Cozolino continues, the hippocampus, temporal lobes, and lateral prefrontal lobes begin to organize the systems of explicit memory. In typically developing children, implicit and explicit memory systems are woven seamlessly together to create a unified conscious experience of the world. With severe trauma, memory systems can become "dissociated," resulting in disturbances of cognition, emotion, and the development of stress-induced trauma. When implicit memory is unconscious, it cannot be thought about and can only be demonstrated via attitudes, beliefs, and behaviors. Thus, children who suffer early adverse childhood experience may enter their school-age years agitated, aggressive, and destructive, engaging in fights, property damage, or animal torture. What is extremely important in the case of IAPI children is that their behavior cannot be experienced as a reaction to a negative past event due to the absence of an explicit memory of the trauma. Rather, it is understood as a natural part of the self and an indication of his or her essential "badness," which is usually reinforced by an array of critical adults and feelings of shame that consolidate into a negative self-image. These experiences are themselves forms of implicit memory: what the mind forgets, the central nervous system (CNS) remembers in the form of fear, pain, and physical maladies (Van der Kolk, 2014).

Post-Adoption Traumatic Experience in the Adoptive Family and at School

Is adoption (the event and the process) trauma producing or trauma reinforcing for a child? Is at least some maladjustment among IAPI children a consequence of the psychologically adverse experience related to adoption itself and the child's adoptive status?

An adoption process in most cases originates from two traumatic events: a child's abandonment in some foreign country and an existence of a childless family in the accepting country (infertility in perspective adoptive parents accounts for the majority of international adoptions). Thus an adoption process involves, along with positive feelings, grief, fear of uncertainty, and identity and attachment problems in the adoptee and the adoptive parents. Both sides in this adoption process are vulnerable and at risk for emotional strain and behavioral collapse. Depending on their age, children may demonstrate a full range of emotional and behavioral issues, at least during the acute adjustment period, which usually takes from several weeks to several months after being involved in such a stressful event.

Studies that have addressed subjective acceptance of adoption by adoptees indicate that although the majority of adopted children view adoption favorably, a significant number of them may experience stress associated with their status as an adopted member of the family. The category of "internationally adopted" may include the negative connotation of being "different," "inferior," "foreign," etc. There is a several-decades long debate about "adopted child syndrome" (Smith, 2001; Baden & O'Leary Wiley, 2007) that includes problems in bonding, low self-esteem, identity crisis, anxiety, and feelings of grief and rejection. The extent to which "adopted child syndrome" accounts for the variance in adoptees' behavioral problems is unknown, but a number of mental health professionals admit that the status of an adopted child can affect the attitude and behavior of an international adoptee (Whitten & Weaver, 2010).

On the other side of the spectrum, some adoptive parents have unrealistically high expectations for IAPI children's school achievements and behavior, which may account for some behavioral difficulties as well (Peters, Atkins, & McKay, 1999). These adoptive parents were described on teachers' questionnaires as "anxious about school results" and as paying "a lot of attention to their children's schoolwork" (Zill, 2017). As noted by Zill, chronic feelings of not being able to satisfy parental standards may be an important stress factor in the adopted child's development.

A number of research publications showed that the type of caregiving environment into which a child is placed after adoption is a determining factor (in addition to the pre-adoption adverse experience) for the severity of maladjustment: an adoptive family's impaired reciprocal relation with an IAPI child is a definite cause of a child's behavior problems (Keys et al., 2008). Thus parental discipline practices and supervision skills have been linked to aggression (Miller, Chan, Tirella, & Perrin, 2009). Such family relationship characteristics as family cohesion, the emotional closeness felt among family members, or, just the opposite, a lack of intra-family communication and support have been found highly predictive of positive or disruptive behavior. There is no reason to expect that adoptive families would be immune from the same parental and family difficulties that have been identified in nonadoptive families. And still, adoptive and biological parents may differ in their expectations of parenting or their children's behavior.

A finding made by Warren (1992) almost three decades ago regarding the referral bias as a factor in statistical significance of prevalence of behavior problems in adopted adolescents is still valid. Warren examined epidemiological data of a national sample of 3,698 adolescents, of whom 145 were adopted. She found that adopted adolescents were referred for psychiatric treatment more often than non-adopted adolescents, regardless of problem severity. Higher referral rates occur even after adjustments for social-economic status (SES) and education of adoptive parents. Adopted adolescents were younger upon admission and were admitted with less severe symptomatology (e.g., higher rates of adjustment disorder vs. lower rates of psychotic disorder). These findings suggest that the proportionately high psychiatric referral rate among adoptees is not attributable entirely to the severity of their behavior problems and is supportive of a referral bias among adoptive parents. At least three explanations of such a "referral bias" suggested by Peters et al. (1999, p. 1): 1) lower threshold for referral among adoptive parents, 2) adoptive parents' higher SES and greater comfort with social service agencies, and 3) adoptive parents' greater concern about family cohesion and lower tolerance for misbehavior.

Unfortunately, post-adoption traumatic experiences related to school functioning are not a focus of most research literature in the field of international adoption. Nevertheless, school is a major frustrating factor that powerfully contributes to the after-adoption traumatic development. Schooling is the leading activity for children aged 5 to 18. For those international adoptees older than 5, the formal schooling begins or continues soon after arrival. Entering our educational system for many international adoptees means nothing less than the beginning of new ongoing stress. The majority of them are not ready to benefit from our school scheme cognitively, socially, academically, or language-wise. Academic failures go hand in hand with social letdowns: children are judged by their peers based on their advancement or a lack of it in school academic and social activities; children form self-image and self-confidence based on their ability to cope with schoolwork; children forge alliances/friendships that are affected by their standing among classmates. Peer rejection sets in and becomes another powerful trauma-producing factor for many IAPI children in post-adoption social situations of development.

Survival Behavior Patterns as a Direct Consequence of Developmental Trauma Disorder

Survival skills include constant alertness and readiness to react to danger, specific means of coping with threats (fighting, fleeing, or dissociation), and certain "special" social skills (manipulation, proactive aggressiveness, triangulation, indiscriminate friendliness to strangers, etc.). Survival skills of an orphanage resident develop early on and dominate their psychological profile. Survival skills forcefully substitute for age-appropriate adaptive skills and patterns of behavior that are not needed for immediate survival, such as academic learning skills, high-order reasoning, and positive socialization skills. Traumatic events in IAPI children's lives are often unpredictable; therefore, a child becomes accustomed to being vigilant in the face of uncertainty, which leads to a fear of change in routines, new situations, and unfamiliar faces. It is to be stressed that survival skills, being repeated numerous times, are deeply embedded into a child's psyche and operate mostly beyond the child's conscious awareness. Once adaptive, while the child was in a stressful dysfunctional family or in an institution, survival behavior patterns cause disruptions in the adoptive family's functioning and in overall post-adoption environment. Survival skills may impede developmental capability to meet societal expectations in learning, self-regulating emotions, interpersonal interaction, cognitive functioning, and other age-appropriate competencies (read more about survival skills in the section titled "Post-Orphanage Behavior (POB) Syndrome").

Mixed Maturity as a Direct Consequence of Developmental Trauma Disorder

It is difficult to pinpoint exactly when and by whom the term "mixed maturity" was first used, but I attribute its origin to Dr. P. Cogen (2008), who used it extensively in her well-known book in the adoptive community titled *Parenting Your Internationally Adopted Child*. The essence of this phenomenon is that the victims of DTD may demonstrate the behavior of an older child and at times of a much younger one. For example, in terms of self-care, alertness to the environment, and basic survival skills, post-institutional children may be well advanced for their age, but in reaction to stress and frustration, they may act like a child several years younger. Their experiences and knowledge of the "dark" side of life could be way above their age expectations and thus shocking to their parents. At the same time, their reactions to social events, interpersonal relationships, academic learning, and their overall adaptive behavior are often so immature that it puzzles and upsets their adoptive parents and teachers. As a result of "mixed maturity," it is difficult for IAPI children to interact with peers, to share interests, to participate in conversation, or to engage in play, sports, or learning activities. Due to their "mixed maturity," they may be isolated in Scout groups, excluded from different spontaneous "projects," and left out during parties. "Mixed maturity" is one of the most confusing characteristics of older IAPI children for parents, teachers, and therapists. We are all conditioned to perceive behavior according to certain socially acceptable norms, so when a 9-year-old boy behaves like a 3-year-old toddler, it is bewildering, to say the least. The adults are prone to respond inconsistently to the adopted child with mixed maturity, thereby validating the child's internal model of the world as unpredictable.

"Mixed maturity" as a psychological phenomenon in **"older" adoptees** may be a product of a peculiar combination of rigid routine with ongoing uncontrollable changes in a typical environment of the overseas institutions: constant turnover of caregivers and frequent transfers of children between and/or within institutions create unpredictability in living arrangements and lead to a tremendous sense of instability and lack of control. On the other hand, children's everyday routines are fixed by rigid schedules with virtually no personal choices. As a result of this everyday routine combined with sudden uncontrollable change, there is a minimal need for behavioral self-regulation, long-term planning, or a need to practice goal-directed consistent behavior. The orphanage residents live in a "reactive" mode, surviving "one day at a time." Immaturity in self-regulation behavior and emotions, the core of the "mixed maturity" phenomenon, can be seen in such behavior patterns as follows:

- These children have difficulty with sustaining goal-directed behavior, independent generation of problem-solving strategies and methods toward achieving goals, carrying out multistep activities and following complex instructions, and monitoring and keeping track of performance outcomes.
- They are emotionally volatile—lacking the ability to modulate emotional responses. These children, whether happy or sad, are easily aroused emotionally; the speed and intensity with which they move to the extremes of their emotions is much greater than that of their same-aged peers; they are often on a roller coaster ride of emotions. As observed by one parent, "When my 8-year-old is happy, he is so happy that people tell him to calm down. When he is unhappy, he is so unhappy that people tell him to calm down."
- They are reluctant or unwilling to perform tasks that are repetitive, uninteresting, require effort, or that they did not choose (but that is what life in general and school learning in particular consist of). It is very hard for them to shift (to make transitions, change focus from one mind-set to another, switch or alternate attention) and to inhibit, resist, or not act on an impulse, including an ability to stop one's activity at the appropriate time.
- These children have difficulty with delaying gratification and accepting "no" for an answer. In this respect, many post-institutionalized children are rather similar to much younger children than to their peers.

These characteristics of immature self-regulation, which, being a part of post-orphanage behavior, may appear as symptoms of ADHD and other neurologically based disorders.

Distorted Attachment as a Direct Consequence of Developmental Trauma Disorder

The security of attachment bonds is the most important alleviating factor against trauma-induced behavior and emotional troubles. Our scientific understanding of the bonding between a parent and a child dates back to the seminal observations of John Bowlby: he postulated that humans are predisposed to seek and sustain relationships that satisfy an intrinsic need for security and perform the important biological function of ensuring the child's protection and survival. Bowlby labeled this process attachment. The failure to develop a secure attachment in infancy appears to reverberate throughout an individual's life in the form of difficulties with relationships and regulation of emotions and impulses. Indeed, in infancy and early childhood, the quality of attachment is the single most important factor that can predict problems later in life (Cozolino, 2014). Bowlby developed the concepts of attachment schema, proximity seeking, and a secure base. His work highlighted the importance of both physical contact and consistent presence of caretakers (Bowlby, 1988). Although not without its critics, Bowlby's attachment theory is today a dominant approach to understanding early social development. It provides us with understanding of the long-term effects of early social-emotional and relationship deficiencies experienced by most institutionalized children.

IAPI children are an extreme group of attachment deprivation: international adoption brought a new dimension to this issue. Let us take two groups of IAPI children who were adopted from the former Soviet Union republics and China. These children constitute roughly half of all international adoptees in the Western countries.

According to the medical records contained in BGCenter database, a staggering 43% of adopted children from Russia were abandoned ("refused at birth" in Russian terminology) in the maternal ward immediately after birth. The regular procedure in Russian children's hospitals is to keep these children in an intensive care unit for three months and then place them in the so-called Baby House (state-run orphanages for babies ages 3 months through 3 years). However, medical history records in our database indicated that the majority of "refused" children spent from 5 to 7 months in an intensive care unit due to severe health problems related to after-birth conditions. The intensive care unit is typically a hospital section that contains several rooms where these children are housed, fed through bottles, and provided with treatment and care from medical personnel who are scheduled to work at a certain time. The notion of "attachment" is just not applicable to this situation.

In the China group, the majority of children were "found" by authorities at railroad stations, on the steps of police headquarters, and at the entrance of hospitals or orphanages. The date of birth is usually assigned based on an educated guess by a medical staff who initially examined the child. In the majority of cases in our database, these children were located by the authorities in the first three months of life. After that, some children spent time in a local hospital, but some were placed immediately in an orphanage. Again, no elements of "attachment" were present for at least the first several months of these children's lives.

Attachment theory consistently showed in numerous contemporary research publications that a lack of a caregiver-child responsive social/emotional interactions is a major contributor to distorted and delayed development, evident in later behavior problems, impaired social skills, etc. According to a number of scientific publications, the most damaging effect is produced within the first 24 to 36 months of life, which seemingly is a sensitive period for forming the base of social connectedness (Landry, Smith, Swank, & Guttentag, 2008; Bruce et al., 2009).

Post-Orphanage Behavior Syndrome

The psychological effects of living in an orphanage on a child's post-adoption behavior did not attract the attention of the general public and scientists in North America until the first waves of international adoptees from Romania hit the US, Canada, and Western Europe in late 1980s. No wonder: in most receiving countries, orphanages were closed several decades before, and the notion of "orphanage behavior" disappeared from the researchers' radar. But when the adoption of children from overseas orphanages reached large numbers, the monster came back unrecognized. It was given many fancy names, like "institutional autism" or "impaired attachment." In fact, it was a pattern of learned survival skills, produced and/or magnified by an early childhood trauma.

It is convincingly shown in many research publications that institutional care is the breeding ground for specific behavior among children who were deprived proper adult mediation in their early most formative years, were continuously traumatized, and were forced into survival mode of everyday life. Post-orphanage behavior (POB) syndrome is a cluster of learned behaviors that could have been adaptive and effective in orphanages but became maladaptive and counter-productive in the post-adoption family, school, and social environment.

Life in a dysfunctional family, on the streets, and later in an institution leads to the formation of the corresponding and somewhat adequate for these hazardous settings behavior patterns known as "orphanage behavior" (Gindis, 2005). These patterns of behavior and a matching "internal model of the world" become the integral part of a child's psychological profile. The new social situation of development (SSD) after the adoption contradicts the existing internal representation and patterns of orphanage behavior. However, children are not robots that we can switch from one pattern of behavior to the other: they continue at least for some time with the survival mode of conduct that served them well in their pre-adoption life. As a result of collision of the child's learned and interiorized orphanage behavior and the demands of a new SSD, the condition of a trauma-producing state is formed: the IAPI child may not be accepted by peers, fails in school, and suffers from the ongoing conflicts in the adoptive family. The new layer of trauma forms and consolidates, being reinforced by a lack of communicative capacity and appropriate cultural background.

The following is a clinical description of behavior observed and reported in IAPI children. Some of these behavior patterns are presented in research literature and some are my generalization based on three decades of clinical work with IAPI children and may need further empirical verification and scientific validation. Please also note that some antisocial acts, such as stealing, habitual lying, or hoarding are also a part of POB syndrome in some children, but due to the clearly pathological nature and relatively limited presentation, these are not discussed here.

Controlling and Avoiding Behavior

Controlling and avoiding behavior is a consequence of a global sense of insecurity typical for many IAPI children. It takes different forms in school and at home. In school, with their fragile and vulnerable sense of competence, former orphanage residents feel that it is better to be perceived as being uncooperative rather than an incompetent underachiever. Being insecure and too sensitive to failure, these children tend to avoid classroom assignments or activities that they perceive as "difficult," hence their refusal or noncompliance. It can be open defiance or hidden sabotage, but it is rooted in their overwhelming need to always be in control, to be on known and manageable "turf." This is an obstacle in their learning: to be a good learner means to take risks, to step into unknown territory, to be sure of one's own ability to cope, and to be prepared to accept help from adults or more competent peers, if and when it is needed.

The early childhood experiences of deprivation and insecurity force a post-institutionalized child to fight for control at home. This fight may assume ugly forms and can be very upsetting for the parents. A substantial part of controlling and avoiding behavior comes from separation anxiety that may be a bizarre form of fear of being sent back to the orphanage, being passed to another family, or just being left alone again in the midst of a totally unknown and hostile environment. For a long time, this fear stays in the minds of many international adoptees in spite of verbal assurances of their adoptive parents, and it may interfere with normal functioning in the family.

Self-Soothing and Self-Stimulating Behavior

A consistent state of neglect of basic emotional needs "educates" orphanage residents on how to take care of their own emotional needs with self-soothing and self-stimulating behavior, which might have been copied from other children or arrived at independently by a child. These might include

- withdrawal/aloofness with finger sucking, hair twisting, full-body spinning and rocking, head spinning and banging, and covering ears to block out even ordinary sounds;
- active resistance to any changes in routine and environment;
- excessive reaction to even ordinary stimuli or unusual reaction to some sensory stimuli (taste, smell, touch);
- making unusual or animal-like sounds for a long time; or
- extreme restlessness or obsessive touching of self and objects.

These patterns of behavior are observed to a different degree in many IAPI children and may decrease or increase in intensity and at times be completely eliminated, but then suddenly reappear in several years. For some professionals and parents, these behaviors may appear as genuinely autistic.

Hyper-Vigilance and "Proactive" Aggressiveness

Children who are neglected and traumatized during early formative years tend to display higher levels of aggressive behavior. "Hyper-arousal," a heightened alertness and vigilance, combined with the inability to correctly interpret the emotional context of the situation, is typical for many post-orphanage children, and it often results in inadequate social interactions, both with peers and adults. Perceived threats can objectively be typical day-to-day events, such as a new environment, loud redirection, the mother's simple request to clean up the room, disrupted routine, or perceived rejection by peers. In such situations, both boy and girl IAPI children can be "tough" and proactively aggressive in their urge to dominate peers and protect themselves from the "expected" hostility of their environment.

Feeling of Entitlement

Due to the very nature of orphanage life, when "goods and services" come from "out of the blue" and are delivered seemingly evenly to everyone in the group, it produces a feeling of entitlement in the orphanage inmates. The dictionary defines "entitle" as "to furnish with a right or claim to something." Entitlement is a normal stage of human development: when an 18-month-old demands possession of everything he sees, it is a natural and passing stage of growth. However, for a 9-year-old, it is not appropriate developmentally: a child should have learned by this time to balance taking and giving. A typically developing child of a certain age learns, for example, that toys come as rewards for achievements or as presents given in certain situations like birthdays, holidays, etc., and not just because the "thing" exists and he or she wants to have it. The feeling of entitlement can be seen when a child whines and screams, demanding a new toy she sees on the store shelf, a new pair of sneakers he has seen his classmates wear, or a new cereal just advertised on TV. A child who was raised in an ordinary family may also have a sense of entitlement, of course. But some children raised in orphanages have this feeling on a much greater scale. They are conditioned to the notion that if one member of a group has something (say, is given a pencil or a notebook), other members of the same group are supposed to get the same, too, whether they need it or not. They may not understand the inappropriateness of their demand when a 17-year-old sibling has the privilege of returning home at ten in the evening. A 12-year-old may hysterically request the same privilege for himself. While a sense of entitlement in children raised in families may result from poor parental techniques, such as giving rewards randomly, in orphanage residents this is a survival skill determined by institutional care. As such, it is only one small step away from the feeling of entitlement to obtain things through theft, robbery, or deception.

Extreme Attention Seeking

Adults' attention is a rare and most valuable commodity in an orphanage, and children there fiercely compete for such attention, sometimes through negative behavior: it is better to be punished than ignored. Orphanage residents constantly seek adults' attention, approval, and encouragement. Often, no matter what they do, the motivation is to evoke a reaction from the grown-up, not to solve a problem or achieve some goal. This extreme urge to obtain attention is borderline with pathology. Thus, I often observe in post-institutionalized children what I call "person-oriented" versus "goal-oriented" behavior. For example, during testing, the child is asked to make a block design according to a model presented in a booklet in front of her. However, the girl will not look at the model but will keep looking at me, randomly moving blocks in anticipation of my reaction. As soon as she infers that I am pleased with her performance, she stops her activity, in spite of the fact that her result is not the same as the model. Her motivation is not to accomplish the task but to please the adult and evoke his sympathy and attention. This urge to win an adult's attention and approval is typical for children in general, but in post-institutionalized children, it often reaches extremes at the expense of independent goal-directed activity. It may adversely affect their performance on standardized tests where the examiner's behavior, by definition, is supposed to be "neutral" and "impartial." In such situations, post-institutionalized children may lose interest and motivation to perform: to "achieve" for many of them means to get an adult's attention, not to accomplish the task.

Indiscriminate Friendliness with Strangers

Orphanage-raised children may show indiscriminate and superficial friendliness with strangers, similar to patients with personality disorders. They may behave inappropriately with complete strangers they meet at a party or in a store. In fact, to their adoptive parents' frustration, they may demonstrate more intimate feelings toward strangers than to their parents. It is always a shock to adoptive parents when I explain to them that for an orphanage resident, any and every adult is a potential parent, and this disconcerting attitude may stay with them for many months after the actual adoption. I remember a 7-year-old boy whom I evaluated after more than a year in the adoptive family. On the second day of testing, he leaned over to me and said, "Will you adopt me? I do not like them (meaning his adoptive parents). I'll better stay with you."

Whereas for family-reared children, apprehension about strangers is the norm, for post-institutionalized children, a friendly approach to any adult willing to pay attention may enhance their chances of being cared for and actually promote positive caregiving. However, the adopted IAPI children may present a more complicated picture: even after becoming attached to their adoptive parent, some are simultaneously indiscriminately friendly to strangers, as it was described in a number of publications (Chisholm, 1998; Bruce et al., 2009).

Learned Helplessness

This is clearly a survival skill in its origin: children in orphanages have been conditioned to get more attention from caregivers when they appear helpless: the more independent children are in an institutional environment, the less attention they receive. Some post-institutionalized children have deeply internalized this behavior and manage to appeal to a wide audience with demonstrated helplessness. Many of these children actually have the needed skills or knowledge, but are resistant to any attempt to encourage them to act independently. There is, of course, a genuine need for help, but sometimes the line between learned helplessness and real need may be rather thin.

In conclusion, this roster of clinically observed patterns of behavior in post-institutionalized children may be present either all or in part in the same child and with a wide range of intensity. There are no gender differences in these behaviors, except withdrawal being more typical for girls and aggressiveness being more typical for boys.

After adoption, every child faces the task of transforming orphanage survival skills into functional family and school relationships. The child has to learn new patterns of behavior and new social skills to interact with adults and peers. The time spent in an orphanage sometimes, but not necessarily always, correlates with the intensity of internalized orphanage survival skills and POB syndrome. The range of individual differences here is very broad. In some adopted children, the transformation of social skills and maturation of self-regulation comes naturally with time and practice. In many cases, POB will diminish by itself through observation and participation in family life (social learning) and figuring out the most appropriate and productive behavior. In others, it may go away quickly, but suddenly reappear under stress. In others yet, it takes a long time, great effort, and sometimes special help (counseling or psychotherapy) to get rid of POB.

It is important to realize that POB has shared overt behavioral symptoms with serious mental/emotional disorders. Therefore, those professionals who have no experience with post-institutionalized children may be easily confused and find a host of disorders from ADHD to attachment disorder, to autism spectrum disorder and affective disorders in children who in fact demonstrate POB. On the other hand, POB may mask, be in addition to, and be reinforced by organic and neurologically based genuine disorders, such as bipolar disorder or ADHD. In talking about "learned" behavior, by no means do I discount the possibility that some of these children may have childhood depression, post-traumatic stress disorder, or ADHD. However, it takes time to diminish the effects of POB in order to understand the underlying emotional problems. Hopefully, a skillful clinician is able to recognize the roots of the issue before putting these children on medication or in specialized programs. The question is, how long do parents need to wait for POB to subside before knowing that something is "still not right" and that there is a problem? The rule of thumb is this: POB syndrome has a tendency to recede with time (several months to a year or longer in some cases), while a genuine disorder will stay and may get worse.

The bottom line is that POB is a "learned" behavior: a set of survival skills that are functional and adaptive in the specific milieu of an orphanage. Therefore, the only remedy is to substitute these orphanage survival skills with the newly learned, different, and, at times, opposite behaviors socially acceptable and efficient in the family and wider social environment.

Clinical Case: Nina—The Orphanage Favorite

An 8-year-old girl named Nina had been living in her adoptive family about a year when her adoptive parents requested an appointment. Nina was born in Russia. Her biological father, having been released from prison, showed up in a small Siberian village, raped or coerced a teenage girl who gave birth to a daughter. Soon after, the 17-year-old mother ran away with her newborn. For the next two years, the young mother wandered around with no permanent place to stay and no work. The means of her living remained uncertain, although the worst suspicions were most likely true. She turned into a vagrant and a drunkard, abandoning her toddler daughter for long hours. After the two years that she and Nina were together, always on the move, never assured of their tomorrow, the mother got tired of her burden, dropped the girl off at her distant relatives, and vanished for good.

Nina's new caretakers filed the paperwork for legal guardianship, and the court promptly stripped the mother of her parental rights. Nina stayed with her relatives for about two years, but for a reason not documented, they placed her into a state-run orphanage. Nina stayed in this institution for nearly a year when she was accepted (on a trial basis) by a local family as a candidate for an adoption. However, she was returned to the orphanage after six months: something with the prospective family didn't work out. Whether there were certain circumstances or the relationship simply lacked chemistry, the girl went through yet another rejection.

Then, in what seemed like the end of misfortunes, an American family took the girl out of her orphanage, out of her country, across an ocean to the land where everything was new and strange. That is what I learned from the girls' file: she lived through a chain of abandonments, neglect, and deprivation during the time that constituted her early childhood: from birth to 7 years.

For Nina's new parents—Cindy and Brad—it was a second marriage; both were highly educated professionals with no parental experience. Both were mesmerized by their new daughter: a blue-eyed blonde cutie, a bright Nina among plain Janes. Sensing that power must be coming from a man, the girl ignored Cindy and was clinging to Brad, choosing him as her favorite. At the beginning, Cindy didn't give it much thought, hoping that with time everything was going to settle and sort itself out, but it didn't.

From their first attempt to take Nina to a doctor, they learned that the girl would not let anyone touch her, screaming and spitting and scratching like a wild cat, calming down and sobbing quietly in Brad's arms only after leaving the office. As time went by, Nina became less volatile, but the situation at home didn't get any better. Brad remained the girl's favorite, and she behaved as if her mother didn't exist at all. Only on one or two occasions, when in Toys R Us, did Nina allow Cindy to take her hand, leading her to a shelf and pointing at a dollhouse. A sober voice in the back of her mind was telling Cindy that she was being played but the hope that it could be the turning point or the milestone blinded her judgment. As soon as the toys were paid for, things plunged back to their hostile status quo.

The parents hired a Russian-speaking "nanny," a live-in helper about the same age as Cindy. The parents were happy that Nina felt more at ease with her au pair, who served as a mediator between the girl and her parents. It was clearly the path of least resistance for Nina: why struggle to learn a new language when the nanny translated everything for her? The help of a native-speaking caregiver definitely made life easier for this adoptive family by enabling communication, but it also complicated life immensely in the long run. Placing another female adult between Cindy and Nina led to serious attachment issues. Nina's learning English was blocked, and for the first months at home, she did not make much progress in mastering her new language.

What prompted my encounter with Nina and her parents was the school. Nina was brought home in May, and her new parents decided to wait for the beginning of a new school year, giving Nina a chance to learn some English. Nina willingly went to school on the first day, but on the second day refused to leave the house in her typical explosive fashion. Nina's parents believed that she was afraid to be abandoned. Someone at school suggested shadowing—that is, accompanying Nina to school and staying around with her for a couple of hours first, then for an hour to ease the girl into her new schedule. This tactic did not work. The next three months were a continuous struggle at home and in school, particularly when the "nanny" quit her job. Only a year after the adoption, the parents, a successful and composed couple in full control of their lives, found themselves totally exhausted and appeared in my office.

At 8 years and 4 months, Nina was tall for her age, proportionally built, and quite dazzling looking. I could see how she had charmed her parents in the orphanage. In the office, I saw the troubling signs immediately: Nina ignored her mother and was literally hanging on her father, pressing herself close to him, clutching his hand, and constantly pulling his sleeve for attention. Her parents were concerned that Nina would refuse to communicate with me; however, just the opposite happened: both days of testing, shared/joint interaction, and a play therapy session with our in-office Russian-speaking therapist went smoothly. To the parents' astonishment, the girl looked relaxed and happy.

I started my first parents' briefing with this statement: "As hard as you think your situation is now, the main struggle is ahead, when Nina feels comfortable with the English language."

"We thought it was the other way around. Isn't that when things correct themselves?"

I explained, "Nina is in a survival mode of her existence right now. I am afraid that in a few more months, Nina will be manipulating teachers and beating up children. I wouldn't even exclude a possibility of her climbing onto her teacher's lap and confessing about abuse at home. Already a master of triangulation, imagine what she can do when language is no obstacle but a tool. Parents will be played against teachers, teachers against classmates. It does not mean that you have a sociopath on your hands. This is a little girl who survived what you cannot even imagine. So, she will continue, for some time, to live in this survival mode, all this will not be planned or prepared, but rather instinctive, spontaneous, deeply embedded behavior."

Then I asked, "Can you describe what Nina's orphanage was like?"

"We haven't seen others to make a comparison," Brad said, "but the place looked like what you'd expect from it: regular conditions, regular children. Regular for an orphanage, that is."

"What about Nina's role there?"

The question plucked a good string. As opposed to all controversial subjects touched upon earlier, that was their undeniable triumph. My visitors exchanged proud glances, and Cindy said, "Everyone loved our little girl there! When we were getting ready to leave, they couldn't help crying. The housemothers and nurses were saying in unison how much they loved Nina, how helpful and outgoing she was. The housemother just wouldn't stop hugging her and wishing her the best."

My question about the orphanage wasn't a mere curiosity: knowing the past helps understand the present. The girl was a typical orphanage favorite—a nightmare for adoptive parents.

To begin from afar, people are susceptible to good looks, an attitude defined by a custom-coined expression: beauty privilege. At the gut level, we all, with no exceptions, sympathize with a beauty and shun a beast. That statement remains just as accurate in other countries, cultures, and times. A cute puppy attracts, while an ugly duckling repels. This phenomenon is spot-on when it comes to adoption. As prospective parents visiting an orphanage, Cindy and Brad were instantly drawn to this charming kid with an open smile, blond hair, and blue eyes. Even if there was a shadow of uncertainty, the dimple in her cheek dotted the final "i" with a bang.

But Nina proved to be not only cute but also smart, tuned-into and experienced in survival, which for children is tightly linked to closeness with adults. Little and weak, children can't make it on their own, and securing the protection of a grown-up becomes their goal. The lack of attention equates to defeat and traumatic experience. Having been abandoned multiple times, the importance of attention, security, and protection was paramount for Nina.

What can a child in an orphanage crowd do to secure an adult's attention? When being good fails, being bad succeeds. On that scale, punishment surpasses indifference, a notion as true for a family as it is for an orphanage or school. Biological children, especially in large families are no exception. When obedience flops, unruly behavior gets them what they want. More often than not, tantrums, tears, and wrecked toys are a plea for attention. Back in the orphanage, a child realizes that the best way to increase her share of attention is to become a teacher's favorite. In addition to a close relationship, the position also guaranties better control and longer one-on-one times.

It's quite likely that in the beginning, Nina offered her help intuitively, without realizing the forthcoming benefits. She tried to be the first to finish the task, sat in the front row, and followed directions obediently. Pretty soon, she became the "assistant" to the housemother helping her with the morning routine (to make sure everyone washed, got dressed, and gathered in the hall). "The group is ready!" she reported elatedly and later in the cafeteria got the seat closer to the housemother, was the first to ask for seconds, received a bigger slice of cake.

With time, Nina's status solidified, being reflected in the orphanage staff review (kind of a reference letter from the orphanage):

> *The girl displays willpower, has good organizational skills . . . she gets moody at times . . . she may punch her group mates but is very attentive and respectful of adults. When reprimanded, she withdraws, starts crying, which at times culminates in a hysterical reaction.*

On a larger scale, the girl came to this country from a place where she had already earned certain privileges, and, as every immigrant has experienced, the loss of status delivers one of the most serious blows during the initial period of transition. From being a favorite, Nina plunged to the lowest step of the social ladder. From being the first pupil in the classroom, she felt she became an "outcast" and bluntly refused to be in this position by refusing to attend school at all. Nina's instinct of survival urges her to use the means of enduring that she knew, one of them being triangulation, a technique used to antagonize one group member against another, gaining power with their split (all these techniques being mostly unconscious existing skills rather planned strategies).

A child cannot be reprogrammed with a snap of a finger. I told Nina's parents that they were facing a typical post-orphanage syndrome, when the former "orphanage favorite's" survival radar kept searching for ways to mimic previous accomplishments, and triangulation was one of the most powerful techniques in Nina's arsenal. Granted, her methods were childish, but nevertheless effective. Thus, whenever Nina needed favors or gifts, she could easily bribe her mom with as little as stroking her hand or letting her comb her hair. Almost against their will, the parents found themselves drawn into the situation of bidding to buy their child's love. This insatiable need for attention creates a foundation for insecure attachment. Their fully developed and proven tricks make orphanage favorites difficult for their adoptive families.

PTSD and IAPI Children

PTSD is typically originated in a discrete, traumatic incident rather than an ongoing pattern of repetitive traumatization. PTSD has a set of well-defined manifestations, but none includes developmental characteristics, and it implies the existence of so-called triggers, which are the reminder(s) of traumatic incident(s). In clinical practice, when PTSD can't account for all the symptoms present, other diagnoses are often used to explain additional symptoms (Friedman, Keane, & Resick, 2014).

DTD occurs as a result of a continuous process, possibly comprising multiple discrete incidents. For this reason, such events do not warrant a diagnosis of PTSD because the events were not "imminently life-threatening," a criterion for PTSD in the *Diagnostic and Statistical Manual of Mental Disorders*, fifth edition (*DSM-5*, 2013). From the developmental perspective, neglect and exposure to multiple adverse occurrences have a much more pervasive effect than a single traumatic incident.

Finally, DTD has roots in the pre-birth conditions, while PTSD can happen only after birth. Most importantly, PTSD diagnosis is not developmental by nature: it does not describe the effect on development or physiological maturation of a child. As observed by van der Kolk, PTSD cannot capture the multiplicity of exposures over critical developmental periods (van der Kolk, 2005, p. 293): "*Isolated traumatic incidents tend to produce discrete conditioned behavioral and biologic responses to reminders of the trauma, whereas chronic maltreatment or unavoidable recurring traumatization . . . has pervasive effects on neurobiological development.*"

PTSD is well researched in adults: clinical description and medical diagnostic criteria are presented in current *DSM-5* and ICD-10 publications. Within the last 30 years, significant research has been done on the same condition in children. It was found that PTSD in children and adults, although common in many aspects, has important differences in the clinical picture and the means of recovery from this disorder.

In both adults and children, PTSD symptoms may last for a long time and may include disturbing memories or flashbacks: nightmares and fear of re-experiencing the traumatic event, which cause avoidance behavior (escaping thoughts, feelings, conversations regarding an event), hyper-arousal (hyper-vigilance, exaggerated startle response), and hypo-arousal (withdrawn, depression-like behavior).

PTSD is diagnosed in many internationally adopted post-institutionalized children. Moreover, there is an opinion that all international adoptees have PTSD to some degree (Hoksbergen & Dijkum, 2001; Hoksbergen, Rijk, van Dijkum, & ter Laak, 2004). This view is somewhat speculative, because it is based not on clinical or research data, but rather on the assumption that if institutionalization and previous life in a neglectful and abusive family are so traumatic, it must result in PTSD. However, even hypothetically, this is not accurate, because we know that PTSD is the product of the interplay between the nature of a specific traumatic experience and the psychological makeup of the person experiencing it. In other words, the same experience may lead to PTSD in some individuals but not in others. Vulnerability to PTSD depends on many factors, such as age, previous experiences, general sensitivity, or preexisting medical and psychological conditions.

From educational and mental health perspectives, it is not productive to accept the notion that all former orphanage-raised children have PTSD as part of their psychological makeup. Although it is true that they as a group are more at risk for PTSD than their peers at large, this diagnosis must be made on an individual basis by a trained mental health professional, because the triggers for PTSD reactions in international adoptees may be so diverse and so different from our cultural background that it takes a specialist in psychological issues of international adoption to figure it out. Thus some of the triggers could be as common as a threat of physical punishment: it was reported by many adoptive parents that any action that had even a remote resemblance to corporal punishment could trigger a reaction that can only be explained by previous traumatic experiences. At the same time, some triggers could be rather "exotic," such as the sight of falling snow or the sound of the child's native language.

Once, clients in my office mentioned that, among other problems with their 8-year-old daughter adopted from Russia four years prior, she could not use hot or even warm water, and bathing her was a "big deal" in their family: she cried and screamed every time and looked terrified. At that moment, I was unable to explain this phenomenon, just mentioned casually that it looked like PTSD-type behavior. However, in the evening of the same day, after reviewing the original (Russian) court documents related to adoption and not translated to the adoptive parents, I found that the biological mother of the girl was incarcerated for attempting to kill her baby by throwing her daughter into boiling water. The child was rescued by relatives, the burn marks on her skin were barely noticeable and could not be explained to the adoptive parents; the girl was only 8 months old at the time of the incident. She, of course, did not remember this experience consciously, but her body did remember the trauma, and hot water was a real trigger of PTSD.

As with other behavior issues in IAPI children, it's important to determine which PTSD symptoms are mild, manageable, and probably transitional in nature, and which are threatening symptoms of a long-lasting trouble.

Therapy has been proven effective to treat PTSD in adults, but it is not necessarily so with children, particularly internationally adopted children: any sensible treatment of PTSD via "talking" therapy is based on the person's language ability. This ability is in itself an issue for international adoptees: their limited English (or quickly disappearing native language capacity) may result in their inability to express feelings and verbalize memories, completely blocking PTSD rehabilitation.

ADHD and IAPI Children

Because of their constant state of hyper-arousal, a child with DTD may present patterns of behavior often associated with ADHD, such as difficulty with sustaining attention, restlessness, and impulsivity. There is evidence of high rates of ADHD diagnoses in the IAPI population, reported by parents, teachers, and mental health professionals (see reviews in Miller, 2004; Gunnar & van Dulmen, 2007; Sonuga-Barke, Kreppner, Beckett, Castle, & Colvert, 2007). In fact, according to several research publications, IAPI children are diagnosed with this disorder three to four times more often than their peers in the population at large (Lindblad, Ringback Weitoft, & Hjern, 2009).

The first researcher who attracted attention to this issue was M. Rutter and his group of associates (Rutter, Kreppner, & O'Connor, 2001). They indicated that there was a very high rate of what they called a "hyperactive-inattentive syndrome" in their sample of IAPI children, but they made a point of not calling it ADHD, because the clinical picture did not fit typical ADHD. For example, in the "typical" ADHD population, the overwhelming majority of affected children are boys, while in the adoption sample, boys and girls were equally affected. The researchers expressed concern that IAPI children were being lumped in with and treated like typical ADHD patients when the etiology and symptoms were often different in significant ways.

One study (Loman, 2012) compared the clinical and symptomatic profiles of the 11- to 15-year-old IAPI children with the non-adopted children diagnosed with ADHD (note that the majority of IAPI children in that sample were adopted from Eastern European countries following longer periods of institutionalization). It was found that IAPI children with symptoms of ADHD revealed an elevated disinhibited social behavior and, among males, more distinct impulsivity. In addition to typical ADHD features, the IAPI group had a few unique features usually not found in typical ADHD population, such as PTSD symptomatology and high rates of aggressive behavior. The author stopped short of naming trauma, but listed several trauma-related characteristics among causes of ADHD-like behaviors.

There is a growing understanding (Abrines et al., 2012) that many IAPI children have been misdiagnosed with ADHD when the difficulties (hyperactivity, inattention, behavioral issues) are actually related to trauma. One thing that most orphanage survivors have in common is poor emotional and behavioral self-regulation. Hyperactive, disorganized, and dis-regulated behaviors that are typical for children with ADHD may reflect in internationally adopted children the effect of early childhood trauma facilitated by abnormal environmental factors of orphanage life. Their hyper-arousal is the result of a sensitized neural response stemming from a specific pattern of repetitive neural activation due to recurring traumatizing experiences. Sensitization occurs when this pattern of activation results in an altered, more sensitive neural system. Once sensitized, the same neural activity can be elicited by less intense external stimuli (Perry, 2006). In other words, the traumatic events in early childhood have the capacity to "redefine" the baseline level of the CNSs involved in the stress response. Research suggests that when a child with a history of adverse childhood experience perceives a threat (real or imagined), it reinforces the sensitized neuronal pathways with the result being a heightened fear/stress response. Being constantly tense and easily aroused, IAPI children produce intensely restless behaviors similar to those observed in children with ADHD (Roskam et al., 2013).

In addition to trauma, the ADHD-like behavior in them, at least in part, is due to a lack of modeling, mediating, and assisting, usually provided by caregivers in the family-based upbringing. This is the effect of missing prior adequate social/cultural influences. The emerging new language also plays a critical role in the development of their self-regulation, because it does not allow IAPI children to gain enhanced control over manifestations of their feelings and helps to inhibit impulsive responses.

The clinical picture becomes even more complex when ADHD in international adoptees coexists with anxiety: in the clinical and research community, there is an ongoing debate regarding the diagnostic overlap between ADHD and generalized anxiety disorder (Berlin, Bohlin, & Rydell, 2003; Nemeroff, 2004). In an IAPI child, the ADHD-like condition includes a significant emotional component (e.g.: anxiety) that mediates behavior.

Autistic-Like Post-Orphanage Behavior vs. Genuine Autism in IAPI Children

The term *institutional autism* has emerged with the influx of children born overseas, raised in orphanages, and adopted by the Western families. Several terms have been used interchangeably: *institutionally induced autism* (Federici, 1998), *quasi-autism* (Rutter, 1999, 2001, 2007), *acquired institutional autism* (Miller, 2004), and *post-institutional autistic syndrome* (Hoksbergen et al., 2005). The common meaning behind all these modifiers of the term autism is that children may acquire either an autistic condition or just autistic symptoms due to their early life in orphanages, hospitals, and other similar institutions.

For the sake of clarity, I will use only one term—namely: *institutional autism*. It must be stressed that institutional autism has nothing in common with the phenomenon of *acquired* or *regressive* autism, a concept that has been debated in the medical community for at least the last 20 years. Acquired or regressive autism is a condition in which children develop normally for the first 12 to 18 months of life and then regress into an increasingly wide spectrum of autistic disorders due to damage done to their immune system by a virus; genetic disposition; intrauterine, prenatal, or neonatal stress; or other causes (Baskin, 2004).

Historically, the notion of "autism induced by institution" can be traced to an article by British/American psychiatrist Rene Spitz (1945). Spitz described several patterns of behavior he observed in young children who had been placed in the London Children's Hospital after their parents perished during the Nazi bombardment of London in 1940–1942. In reaction to emotional trauma, loss of primary caregiver, isolation in hospital cribs, and lack of stimulation, these children developed symptoms that were at least similar to those often found in children with autism. The notion of *hospitalism*, invented by Spitz, was not used much over the next 50 years, until the massive adoption from Romanian orphanages by American, Canadian, and British families began in the late 1980s and early 1990s. Almost simultaneously, researchers in Canada, the US, and Western Europe began using the notion of hospitalism and later *institutional autism* in describing young children adopted from Romanian orphanages.

Following in the footsteps of Spitz, the researchers depicted autistic-like behavior in children, seen as a result of the ultimate deprivation and isolation associated with living in an institution. In essence, these authors conveyed that orphans learned autistic patterns of behavior due to their experiences in orphanages: such self-stimulating behavior as rocking, picking at themselves, head banging, withdrawal, limited verbal expression, rituals, and emotional outbursts in response to changes in routine were the ways in which institutionalized children learned to fill the gaps in their lonely and desperate lives. Thus, according to Federici (1998, p. 74), "*Over time they practiced these behaviors as a defense mechanism to block out pain and misery and had ultimately become self-absorbed and withdrawn in a way similar to children with autistic conditions.*"

The prevalence of autism and other developmental disabilities in internationally adopted children is unknown at the moment, although there is a widespread belief that orphanage residents are more prone to developmental disabilities than their peers at large (Miller, 2004; Welsh, Andres, Viana, Petrill, & Mathias, 2007). It is understood that in addition to general risk factors that predispose institutionalized children to any developmental disability (heredity and the neurological makeup of the child), there are secondary factors, social in nature (such as a lack of postnatal care and negative conditions of development in institutions), that facilitate the formation of developmental delays and disabilities in this population. The proportion of *organic* (genuine, biologically based) autism and institutionally induced autistic-like behavior in orphanages residents is also unknown. The only statistical research data at this point are provided by Rutter and his colleagues in their publications, based on relatively small samples, dated 1999, 2001, 2007; Hoksbergen, Laak, Rijk, Dijkum, and Stoutjesdijk (2005).

Rutter (1999, 2001, 2007) and his colleagues examined 165 children adopted from Romania before the age of 4. The children were examined at the years 4, 6, and 12, and compared with 52 children of the same age and gender adopted in infancy in the UK. The researchers found 12% of Romanian adoptees had *quasi-autistic features* (versus none in the UK sample) that included rocking, self-injury, unusual and exaggerated sensory responses, and problems chewing and swallowing. (The study was mostly based on adoptive parents' interviews: the Autism Screening Questionnaire was completed by all participants and the Autism Diagnostic Interview was administered to those parents who reported autistic symptoms.) The investigators found that, with the exception of unusual sensory responses, the rate of autistic-like behaviors in most cases steadily declined after the child entered the adoptive family. In a number of cases, however, the difficulties remained, despite good-quality care in the new home. The longitudinal study of this sample (started at the age of 4) indicated that a quarter of the children who had previously shown autistic-like features were completely free of these symptoms at the age of 12. The authors concluded that although initially the autistic-like patterns of overt behavior were found in over 10% of the sample, after years of living with their adoptive families, the significance of these features was diminished dramatically. The authors (Rutter et al., 2007) stressed (p. 1200) that "although there were important similarities with 'ordinary' autism, the dissimilarities suggest a different meaning."

Unfortunately, no further analysis was provided, and the reader remains with the impression that while some children in the studied group show definite signs of autism, others have something else of an unknown nature that may resemble autism.

Hoksbergen et al. (2005) and his group basically repeated the research design of Rutter's studies and applied it to 80 Romanian children adopted by families in the Netherlands. (Adoptive parents were interviewed using the Autism Diagnostic Interview.) In about one-third of the group, the parents reported (in retrospect, because the children had already lived in the families for four to five years at the time of the interview—BG) stereotypic behaviors and communication and language disorders. Six out of 80 were diagnosed with full-fledged autism, while 7 showed some autistic behaviors (in a relatively mild degree) even 5 years after adoption. As in Rutter's study, there was no statistical difference between the genders (please note that in organic-based autism, males have a higher incidence). Like Rutter, Hoksbergen found that those who had been in their adoptive families for five years or longer showed fewer autistic-like behavior problems than children who had been in their adoptive families less than five years.

One may conclude the following from the Rutter et al. and Hoksbergen et al. studies described earlier:

1. On arrival, a significant number (from 10% to 30% in their samples) of former orphanage residents from Romania presented with patterns of behavior similar to those observed in children diagnosed with autism. These patterns included

    (a) Self-stimulating behaviors (rocking, head banging, shaking of hands, face shielding),
    (b) Self-mutilating behaviors (hair pulling, picking at the body),
    (c) Abnormal responses to sensory stimulation (seeking unusual tactile sensations, attraction to bright visual stimulation),
    (d) Temper tantrums in response to change in routine and seemingly unmotivated uncontrollable outbursts of rage and aggression, and
    (e) Some behaviors that are normally not associated with autism (e.g., problems chewing and swallowing).

2. In contrast to organic-based autism, in which boys are more affected, the listed behaviors were equally present in both genders.
3. These patterns are mostly evident upon arrival, and most symptoms diminish in intensity and usually disappear the longer the children are with their adoptive families.
4. A minority of children continue to exhibit these difficult behavior patterns for many years. Thus, in Hoksbergen's study, 7.5% of the children in his sample were diagnosed with autism, while the usual prevalence in the population at large is less than 1%, according to *DSM-5*.

Based on the review of a short list of existing publications on institutional autism, the question can be raised of whether this notion reflects clinical reality. In the samples studied by Rutter and Hoksbergen, there were two categories of children: those who had genuine autism and those who demonstrated a rather heterogeneous cluster of behaviors, with some patterns similar to those observed in truly autistic children. Both the nature and the psychological mechanism of these *autistic-like* behaviors remain unexplained. In addition, none of the reviewed publications discussed a crucial element in producing autistic-like behavior—namely, abrupt native language attrition (Gindis, 1999, 2005). Indeed, practically all international adoptees experience the process of speedy native language loss and the relatively slow process of new language learning, which may heavily contribute to autistic-like behavior during the initial adjustment period when institutional autism is mostly observed.

The BGCenter clinical database contains the results of 389 cases of screenings upon arrival of IAPI children who demonstrated autistic-like behavior. These evaluations were performed within the first 2 to 10 weeks of the children's arrival in the USA. All assessments were done in the children's native language (the children were adopted mostly from the countries of Eastern Europe, republics of the former Soviet Union, Guatemala, and China). The ages in our sample ranged from 3 years 6 months to 9 years 6 months. The purpose of screening upon arrival was to check for possible mental health issues, to facilitate appropriate school placement, and to determine the need for mental health or school-based remedial services. Screening consisted of cognitive, language, adaptive behavior, and academic readiness components (see Addendum 2 for more details). A thorough parent interview included an inventory of autistic behavior in their children using the Children Autism Rating Scale (CARS). The screening was done during the acute phase of the child's initial adjustment to the family and the new social/cultural environment. Indeed, many parents reported behaviors (see the following) that were similar to those listed in Rutter's publications. These patterns of behavior, varying in intensity, were mostly transitory, but in some cases, the children persisted in displaying overt autistic symptoms:

1. Self-soothing, which included withdrawal (aloofness) with finger sucking or clothes sucking, hair twisting, full-body spinning and rocking, head spinning and banging, covering ears to block out even ordinary sounds
2. Self-stimulating, including excessive reaction to even ordinary stimuli, extreme restlessness, obsessive touching of self and objects, making weird and animal-like sounds
3. Resistance to any changes in routine and environment
4. Unusual reaction to some sensory stimuli (taste, smell, touch)

There is no gender difference in these behaviors. Also, it is important to note that most often, these behaviors were observed in a younger cohort (3 to 5 years old); however, if these behaviors were found in children older than 5 years old, these patterns were more persistent and in many cases turned out to be symptoms of genuine autism. As reported by our respondents, typically, the dynamic of observed autistic-like behaviors goes from a rather intense degree upon arrival to a relatively rapid loss of intensity and at least partial disappearance within several weeks or months after entering the family.

One common denominator for all these behaviors among international adoptees is a rapid native language attrition. It significantly limits verbal communication during the first several weeks of the child's life in the family, when institutional behavior is at its peak. A lack of or severe limitation in verbal communication typically leads to significant regression in the child's behavior and the emergence of the autistic-like self-stimulating and self-soothing conduct. To the best of my knowledge, no research has been done on the links between the transient autistic symptoms and the language transition experienced by international adoptees within the first several months in an adoptive family. So far, this is a hypothesis that has been born from empirical observations. It is supported, although indirectly, by the finding that children who are adopted within their native countries (that is, do not experience language disruption) have fewer autistic symptoms than international adoptees (Groark, Muhamedrahimov, Palmov, Nikiforova, & McCall, 2005).

Making a differential diagnosis between autism, post-institutional behavior, and temporary patterns of behavior related to the adjustment period and abrupt language attrition is one of the most daunting tasks in the field of mental health and rehabilitation of IAPI children. The verbal communication deficiency during the initial adjustment period, followed by abrupt first-language attrition, provokes patterns of behavior that fit a description of autism very well. In many ways, such abnormal behaviors may be a typical human reaction to a new and unmanageable situation. In addition to testing, the correct diagnosis requires skillful observation, a thorough parent interview, and a study of the child's adoption documentation. A careful review of the developmental history after adoption is crucial because such features of institutional behavior as repetitive self-stimulating, self-soothing, and a lack of the appropriate spontaneous social interactions show dramatic improvement with time, in contrast to symptoms associated with the genuine autistic spectrum disorders.

A major distinguisher between organic-based autism and temporary autistic-like institutional behavior is the presence of a positive dynamic in the child's development in the family. While most behaviors originating in organic-based autism persist, showing only small and slow, if any, changes, the same identifiable behaviors associated with institutional behavior and loss of language should diminish progressively until they completely disappear, although they may resurface in response to stress and environmental challenges. The timetable depends on a child's age and a host of individual differences, but if autistic-like behavior patterns do not diminish in intensity after about six months in the family, it is likely that we are dealing with organic-based autism or another variation of developmental disability.

Another distinguisher is the severity of a problem within a constellation of symptoms. In organic-based autism, the symptoms are usually more clearly defined and presented in well-known clusters described in the professional literature. Institutional behavior reflects only separate patterns of autistic behavior that are not consistent and can often be explained by environmental circumstances.

Based on the information presented, it is likely that in the samples studied by Rutter and by Hoksbergen, both groups (children with organic-based autism and learned orphanage behavior) were present. Those children whose behavior improved with time spent in the family demonstrated temporary orphanage behavior patterns, whereas those with stubborn autistic symptoms most likely had organic-based autism.

A differential diagnosis between difficulties in initial adjustment, post-institutional behavior, and autism has significant practical implications, as both may have similar overt behavior patterns, and both may be present in internationally adopted children, but these conditions require entirely different remedial approaches. The notion of institutional autism is confusing for personnel involved in remedial work with post-institutionalized children because, if a child has autism, a range of proper educational remedial methodologies and administrative placement and services should take place. If a child demonstrates temporal adjustment difficulties and post-institutional behavior, a completely different set of actions should be considered. The notion of institutional autism gives false hope to adoptive parents, leading them to believe that their children will outgrow autism, which is a severe neurologically based medical condition. As a result, the notion of "institutional autism" may divert the parents' efforts and de-mobilize them in their search for an appropriate remedial program for their children.

In contrast to autism, institutional behavior is the product of specific social conditions, is to be recognized as a learned maladaptive behavior, and should be addressed with behavior modification methodologies commonly used for non-autistic children. One time-tested recommendation is that children with institutional behavior should not be placed in the same programs as children with organic-based autism to prevent their mimicking and reinforcing inappropriate behaviors. Parental consultation and counseling, modification of parenting techniques, changing parental expectations and attitudes, using short-term behavior programs, and addressing specific behavior have proven to be effective in addressing issues of institutional behavior.

The biological nature of autism is well documented (Freitag, 2007), suggesting that social factors (e.g. "*deep institutional privation*" as coined by Rutter, 1999) without known neurological aberration (or other biological and genetic causes) can result in autism (even with modifiers such as *institutional*) seems a relic of psychogenic theories of the causes and origins of autism. It is a scientific fact that no known psychological factors in a child's development have been shown to cause autism, and autism spectrum disorders are certainly not caused by bad parenting or rearing in an institution. *Institutional autism* is merely a confusing metaphor; instead of using this misleading term, a differential diagnosis is the first step in crafting a solution.

Attachment Disorder in IAPI Children: Putting Square Pegs in the Round Holes

I already listed attachment issue as one of the major consequences of DTD in IAPI children. In my clinical experience, the diagnosis of AD is one of the most complex and controversial in the field of international adoption.

For adoptive parents, there is no more emotionally charged issue than attachment. No wonder—attachment is the core of adoption, and failed attachment ruins the very nature of adoption. Attachment difficulties, and their extreme known as attachment disorder, mean an inability to form and maintain age-appropriate intimate relationships within the family. Little is known about the biological causes of this condition, and a mainstream understanding is that attachment disorder is due to pathological care—that is, a disregard for the child's basic emotional needs for security, comfort, stimulation, and affection in the early and most formative years.

The American Psychiatric Association in its *DSM-5* (2013) defines reactive attachment disorder (*DSM-5* code 313.89) with three criteria (pp. 265–266).

A. *A consistent pattern of inhibited, emotionally withdrawn behavior towards adult caregivers.*

B. *A persistent social and emotional disturbance characterized. . . . by minimal social and emotional responsiveness, limited positive effect, episode of unexplained irritability, sadness, or fearfulness.*

C. *The child has experienced a pattern of extremes of insufficient care as evidenced by . . . social neglect or deprivation . . . including . . . rearing in unusual settings that severely limit opportunities to form selective attachments, e.g., institutions with high child-to-caregiver rations.*

As seen from the definition, AD stems from unusual early experiences of systematic neglect and deprivation of the child's basic physical and emotional needs. It could happen because of abrupt separation from caregivers or a lack of caregiver responsiveness to the child, or frequent change of caregivers. All the aforementioned are typical for children in overseas orphanages and make them "at risk" to have or to be at least predisposed to developing AD. It is no wonder that there is a widespread opinion that attachment issues are to be found in all international adoptees, and we can talk only about the degree of this disorder (Bakermans-Kranenburg et al., 2011). At first glance, it makes sense: practically all internationally adopted post-orphanage children come to adoptive homes after experiencing what is defined earlier as "pathogenic care." Real life, however, is more complex than the theory: pathogenic care must meet with certain personality qualities to result in AD.

Like many other psychological conditions, AD ranges from severe to mild, from incurable to a transient and minor state. Some children are damaged beyond their ability to form a connection. Others bond almost instantly and forever. But most of the time, the readiness to form an attachment to newly acquired parents and siblings is somewhere in between. Attachment is a behaviorally defined phenomenon: no litmus paper or laboratory test can detect it. Based on the observed patterns of behavior and relationships, a competent professional could determine whether AD exists as well as the degree of disturbance.

Attachment issues and AD are realities that profoundly affect the lives of many people. Unfortunately, AD has become a scapegoat often being over diagnosed in the international adoption community. Internationally adopted children have been a mystery for parents and professionals, who often can't understand their behavior and motivation, thus prompting a search for a "simple" explanation. And such an explanation in the early '90s became an "attachment." Unfortunately, AD is often used as a "catchall term" to cover a range of different behaviors. Here are only two examples of the "laundry list" of symptoms attributed to AD:

Hughes (2003) defines major characteristics of AD as "*aggression, dissociation, affect and behavioral disregulation, impulsivity, alterations in consciousness, loss of meaning, somatization, inability to differentiate facial expressions, lack of eye contact with caregivers, discomfort with touch, shame*" (p. 271).

Coleman (2003) suggested these features of AD: "*Physical aggression, emotionally deficient social behavior, tantrums, recklessness, risk taking, bullying, stealing, abuse of pets, hoarding food, deception, emotional insatiability, need to control others, defiance*" (p. 205).

The aforementioned seems like an eclectic pileup that belongs to different psychiatric disorders. To complicate matters even more, AD is often mixed up with the learned POB and confused with normal initial adjustment in an adoptive family. Some professionals, particularly those specializing in AD, tend to interpret any symptom in the AD context, following the famous maxima, "If your only tool is a hammer, everything becomes a nail."

However, according to the American Psychiatric Association Position Statement approved by the Board of Trustees in June 2002 (APA, 2002),

> *Reactive Attachment Disorder (RAD) is a complex psychiatric condition that affects a small number of children. The child with RAD may appear detached, unresponsive, inhibited or reluctant to engage in age-appropriate social interactions. Alternatively, some children with RAD may be overly and inappropriately social even with strangers. The social and emotional problems associated with RAD may persist as the child grows older.*
>
> (p. 1)

Particularly frustrating is when children with autistic spectrum disorder are labeled with AD. The two conditions are incompatible; a person with autism cannot have AD by definition (Mercer, 2006; Murin, Willis, Minnis, Mandy, & Skuse, 2011). I have often met children in my practice with autism spectrum disorder (sometimes not properly identified) who spent years in attachment therapy to end up with the parents and child growing frustrated. In my clinical experience, two other occurrences, namely, learned "orphanage survival skills" and behavior during an acute adjustment period are major producers of behavioral patterns that may be mistakenly taken as symptoms of AD.

I believe that internationally adopted children are grossly overdiagnosed with attachment issues in particular when language and cultural components of behavior are ignored and POB and difficulties in the adjustment process are interpreted as attachment failure symptoms. It takes time, observation, and professional help to determine the presence of AD as a part of other disorders or differentiate it from other conditions with similar symptoms.

Initially, adoptive parents and their children meet as strangers, and it would be a miracle if any internationally adopted children were completely attached to adoptive parents upon arrival or even within the first several months. Attachment is a two-way street: attachment from parents to a child and from a child to his or her adoptive parents. It is unfair morally and unproductive clinically to place the burden on a child and focus on forcing him/her to develop the bond. Unfortunately, rather than moving toward one another, some parents expect their adopted children to do the adjusting.

In practice, it may take a long time of slow progression until the final realization that the attachment is not going to form. The reasons for this may become apparent only years later: initial language barrier, inappropriate parental techniques, deep-seated developmental trauma disorder, depression in a parent, strong disagreement in the family, and many other causes, often combined and thus facilitating each other.

Attachment in many aspects is a learned social behavior for a child as well for his or her adoptive parents. Every process of attachment is individual; every child and every parent will have to make adjustments (Coleman, 2003). The bonding varies as much as personalities differ. Paraphrasing Leo Tolstoy, happy families with attachment are all alike; every family with attachment difficulties is unhappy in its own way.

Concluding this chapter, I have to point out that the consequences of DTD reveal themselves in many forms and shapes: behavior is an emergent property of the nervous system, driven by environment and experience, and resulting in both internal and external initiated actions and reactive responses (National Scientific Council on the Developing Child, 2004). Chronic re-experiencing of trauma, a survival model of behavior, "mixed maturity" in social interactions and adaptive behavior, rigidity of behavior resulting in POB syndrome—all these overt behavior patterns manifest themselves in a complex mosaic of factors that cause behavior issues in IAPI children. Due to a combination of neurological and social factors, internationally adopted post-institutionalized children are diagnostically complicated, and their clinical picture is often not consistent with any diagnostic entity. Indeed, simultaneous coexistence of several medical and psychological conditions is common in this population, and a differential diagnosis is crucial for their proper educational remediation and medical and psychological treatment.

References

Abrines, N., Barcons, N., Marre, D., Brun, C., Fornieles, A., & Fumado, V. (2012). ADHD-like symptoms and attachment in internationally adopted children. *Attachment and Human Development, 14*(4), 405–423.

American Psychiatric Association. (2002). *Reactive attachment disorder position statement.* Retrieved from www.psych.org/archives/200205.pdf

American Psychiatric Association. (2013). *Diagnostic and statistical manual of mental disorders* (5th ed.). (DSM-5). Washington DC: APA.

Baden, A. L., & O'Leary Wiley, M. (2007). Counseling adopted persons in adulthood: Integrating research and practice. *The Counseling Psychologist, 35,* 868–901.

Bakermans-Kranenburg, M. J., Steele, H., Zeanah, C. H., Muhamedrahimov, R. J., Vorria, P., Dobrova-Krol, N. A., . . . Gunnar, M. R. (2011). Attachment and emotional development in institutional care: Characteristics and catch-up. *Monographs of the Society for Research in Child Development, 76*(4), 6291.

Baskin, D. (2004). *Presentation to the immunization safety review committee.* Washington, DC: The National Academies Press.

Berlin, L., Bohlin, G., & Rydell, A. (2003). Relations between inhibition, executive functioning, and ADHD symptoms: A longitudinal study from age 5 to 8 1/2 years. *Child Neuropsychology, 9,* 255–266.

Bowlby, J. (1988). Attachment, communication, and the therapeutic process. *A Secure Base: Parent-Child Attachment and Healthy Human Development,* 137–157.

Bruce, J., Tarullo, A. R., & Gunnar, M. R. (2009). Disinhibited social behavior among internationally adopted children. *Development and Psychopathology, 21,* 157–171.

Chisholm, K. (1998). A three-year follow-up of attachment and indiscriminate friendliness in children adopted from Romanian orphanages. *Child Development, 69,* 1092–1106.

Cogen, P. (2008). *Parenting your internationally adopted child.* Boston, MA: The Harvard Common Press.

Coleman, P. K. (2003). Reactive attachment disorder in the context of the family: A review and call for further research. *Emotional and Behavioural Difficulties, 8,* 205–216.

Colvert, E., Rutter, M., Beckett, C., Castle, J., Groothues, C., & Hawkins, A. (2008). The delayed onset of emotional difficulties following severe early deprivation: Findings from the ERA study. *Development and Psychopathology, 20,* 547–567.

Cozolino, L. (2014). *The neuroscience of human relationships: Attachment and the developing social brain* (2nd ed.). New York: W.W. Norton and Co.

Federici, R. (1998). *Help for hopeless child: A guide for families.* Alexandria, VA: Federici & Associates.

Freitag, C. (2007). The genetics of autistic disorders and its clinical relevance: A review of the literature. *Molecular Psychiatry, 12*(1), 2–22.

Friedman, M. J., Keane, T. M., & Resick, P. A. (2014). *Handbook of PTSD: Science and practice* (2nd ed.). New York, NY: Guilford Press.

Gindis, B. (2005). Cognitive, language, and educational issues of children adopted from overseas orphanages. *Journal of Cognitive Education and Psychology, 4*(3), 290–315.

Gleitman, I., & Savaya, R. (2011). Adjustment of adolescent adoptees: The role of age of adoption and exposure to pre-adoption stressors. *Children and Youth Services Review, 33*(5), 758–766.

Groark, C., Muhamedrahimov, R., Palmov, O., Nikiforova, N., & McCall, R. (2005). Improvements in early care in Russian orphanages and their relationship to observed behaviors. *Journal of Infant Mental Health, 26*(2), 96–109.

Grotevant, H. D., & McDermott, J. M. (2014). Adoption: Biological and social processes linked to adaptation. *Annual Review of Psychology, 65*, 235–265.

Gunnar, M., & Van Dulmen, M. (2007). Behavior problems in post-institutionalized internationally adopted children. *Development and Psychopathology, 19*(1), 129–148.

Hawk, B. N., & McCall, R. B. (2011). Specific extreme behaviors of post-institutionalized Russian adoptees. *Developmental Psychology, 47*(3), 732–738.

Hoksbergen, R., & Dijkum, C. (2001). Trauma experienced by children adopted from abroad. *Adoption & Fostering, 25*(2), 18–25.

Hoksbergen, R., Laak, J., Rijk, K., Dijkum, C., & Stoutjesdijk, F. (2005). Post-institutional autistic syndrome in Romanian adoptees. *Journal of Autism and Developmental Disorders, 35*(50), 615–623.

Hoksbergen, R., Rijk, K., van Dijkum, C., & ter Laak, J. (2004). Adoption of Romanian children in the Netherlands: Behavior problems and parenting burden of upbringing for adoptive parents. *Developmental and Behavioral Pediatrics, 25*(3), 175–180.

Hostinar, C., Stellern, S., Schaefer, C., Carlson, S., & Gunnar, M. (2012). Associations between early life adversity and executive function in children adopted internationally from orphanages. *Proceedings of the National Academy of Sciences, 109*, 17208–17212.

Hughes, D. A. (2003). Psychological interventions for the spectrum of attachment disorders and interfamilial trauma. *Attachment and Human Development, 5*, 271–277.

Ji, J., Brooks, D., Barth, R. P., & Kim, H. (2010). Beyond pre-adoptive risk: The impact of adoptive family environment on adopted youth's psychosocial adjustment. *American Journal of Orthopsychiatry, 80*(3), 432–442.

Juffer, F., & van IJzendoorn, M. (2005). Behavior problems and mental health referrals of international adoptees: A meta-analysis. *Journal of the American Medical Association, 293*(20), 2501–2515.

Keys, M., Sharma, A., Elkins, I., Iacono, W., & McGue, M. (2008). The mental health of US adolescents adopted in infancy. *Archives of Pediatrics & Adolescent Medicine, 162*(5), 419–425.

Kreppner, J. M., O'Connor, T. G., & Rutter, M. (2001). Can inattention/ overactivity be an institutional deprivation syndrome? *Journal of Abnormal Child Psychology, 29*, 513–528.

Landry, S., Smith, K., Swank, P., & Guttentag, C. (2008). A responsive parenting intervention: The optimal timing across early childhood for impacting maternal behaviors and child outcomes. *Developmental Psychology, 44*(5), 1335–1353.

Lindblad, F., Ringback Weitoft, G., & Hjern, A. (2010). ADHD in international adoptees: A national cohort study. *European Child Adolescent Psychiatry, 19*, 37–44.

Loman, M. (2012). *Is deprivation-related ADHD different from ADHD among children without histories of deprivation?* University of Minnesota Digital Conservancy. Retrieved from http://hdl.handle.net/11299/138217

Mercer, J. (2006). *Understanding attachment: Parenting, child care and emotional development.* Westport, CT: Praeger Publishers.

Merz, E., & McCall, R. (2010). Behavior problems in children adopted from psychosocially depriving institutions. *Journal of Abnormal Child Psychology, 38*(40), 459–470.

Miller, L. C. (2004). *The handbook of international adoption medicine: A guide for physicians, parents, and providers.* Oxford, UK: Oxford University Press.

Miller, L. C., Chan, W., Tirella, L. G., & Perrin, E. (2009). Outcomes of children adopted from Eastern Europe. *International Journal of Behavior & Development, 33*.

Murin, M., Willis, C., Minnis, H., Mandy, W., & Skuse, D. (2011). *Discriminating reactive attachment disorder from autism spectrum disorders: Key symptoms and clinical characteristics (International society for autism research).* Retrieved from https://imfar.confex.com/imfar/2011/webprogram/Paper9121.html

National Scientific Council on the Developing Child. (2004). *Young children develop in an environment of relationships.* Working Paper No. 1. Retrieved from www.developingchild.net

Nemeroff, C. B. (2004). Neurobiological consequences of childhood trauma. *Journal of Clinical Psychiatry, 65*(1), 18–28.

Perry, B. (2006). Childhood trauma, the neurobiology of adaptation & use-dependent development of the brain: How states become traits. *Infant Mental Health Journal, 16*(4), 271–291.

Peters, B. R., Atkins, M. S., & McKay, M. M. (1999). Adopted children's behavior problems: A review of five explanatory models. *Clinical Psychology Review, 19*(3), 297–328.

Roskam, I., Stievenart, M., Tessier, R., Muntean, A., Escobar, M., Santelices, M., . . . Pierrehumbert, B. (2013). Another way of thinking about ADHD: The predictive role of early attachment deprivation in adolescents' level of symptoms. *Social Psychiatry and Psychiatric Epidemiology, 49*(1), 1–19.

Rutter, M., Andersen-Wood, L., Beckett, C., Bredenkamp, D., Castle, J., & Groothues, C. (1999). Quasi-autistic patterns following severe early global privation. *Journal of Child Psychology and Psychiatry, 40*, 537–549.

Rutter, M., Beckett, C., Castle, J., Colvert, E., Kreppner, J., & Mehta, M. (2007). Effects of profound early institutional deprivation: An overview of findings from a UK longitudinal study of Romanian adoptees. *European Journal of Developmental Psychology, 4*(3), 332–350.

Rutter, M., Kreppner, J. M., & O'Connor, T. G. (2001). Specificity and heterogeneity in children's responses to profound institutional privation. *British Journal of Psychiatry, 179*, 97–103.

Smith, J. (2001). The adopted child syndrome: A methodological perspective. *Families in Society, 82*(5), 491–497.

Sonuga-Barke, E. S., Kreppner, J. M., Beckett, C., Castle, J., & Colvert, E. (2007). Inattention/overactivity following early severe institutional deprivation: Presentation and associations in early adolescence. *Journal of Abnormal Child Psychology, 36*, 385–398.

Spitz, R. (1945). Hospitalism: An inquiry into the genesis of psychiatric condition in early childhood. In *The psychoanalytic study of the child* (Vol. 1, pp. 53–74). New York: International Universities.

Stevens, S. E., Sonuga-Barke, E. S., Kreppner, J. M., Beckett, C., Castle, J., & Colvert, E. (2007). Inattention/overactivity following early severe institutional deprivation: Presentation and associations in early adolescence. *Journal of Abnormal Child Psychology, 36*, 385–398.

Tarullo, A. R., Bruce, J., & Gunnar, M. R. (2007). False belief and emotion understanding in post-institutionalized children. *Social Development, 16*(1), 57–78.

Tieman, W., van der Ende, J., & Verhulst, F. C. (2005). Psychiatric disorders in young adult intercountry adoptees: An epidemiological study. *American Journal of Psychiatry, 162*(3), 592–598.

Van der Kolk, B. A. (2005). Developmental trauma disorder. *Psychiatric Annals,* 401–408.

Van der Kolk, B. A. (2014). *The body keeps the score: Brain, mind, and body in the healing of trauma.* New York: Viking.

Warren, S. B. (1992). Lower threshold for referral for psychiatric treatment for adopted adolescents. *Journal of the American Academy of Child and Adolescent Psychiatry, 31*, 512–527.

Welsh, J., Andres, G., Viana, A., Petrill, S., & Mathias, M. (2007). Interventions for internationally adopted children and families: A review of the literature. *Child and Adolescent Social Work Journal, 24*(3), 285–311.

Whitten, K. L., & Weaver, S. R. (2010). Adoptive family relationships and healthy adolescent development: A risk and resilience analysis. *Adoption Quarterly, 13*(3–4), 209–226.

Wright, L., & Flynn, C. C. (2006). Adolescent adoption: Success despite challenges. *Children and Youth Services Review, 28*, 487–510.

Zill, N. (2017). *The changing face of adoption in the United States.* Publication of Institute for Family Studies. Retrieved from https://ifstudies.org/blog/the-changing-face-of-adoption-in-the-united-states

7 Academic Performance and Educational Remediation of Internationally Adopted Post-Institutionalized Children

Introduction

It is an undeniable fact that in modern societies, schooling (education, training, etc.) is the leading activity for children ages 5 to 18. Moreover, school is an institution in which children get not only an education but also social experience; it's a place where they develop and grow mentally, socially, and emotionally. Children form their self-image and self-confidence based on their ability to cope with school challenges, both academic and social. Schooling, as a leading activity, defines all the other aspects of a child's life, including functioning in the family. School years are expected to be a productive and happy part of a childhood, but in real-life school is often the main source of frustration and stress for a child. Being disruptive, frustrating, or chronically conflicting, the leading activity brings "toxic" stress into a child's existence. Schooling presents additional difficulties for internationally adopted children who are not ready for this experience from many perspectives and are so emotionally fragile that they can be traumatized when pushed by expectations that are beyond their reach. The fact is that too many, if not the majority of, internationally adopted children, despite their resiliency and strong family support, have overwhelming school-related difficulties, and for many of them, school can be qualified as a traumatic experience.

The Overview of Academic Functioning of IAPI Children

A review of an existing body of research related to academic functioning of IAPI children revealed that as a group, they perform way below norms for their grades and age when compared with their non-adopted peers and have substantially more school-related behavior problems (Gindis, 1998, 2006; Dalen, 2001; Dole, 2005; Van IJzendoorn & Juffer, 2006; Beckett, Castle, Rutter, & Sonuga-Barke, 2010; Helder, Mulder, & Linder-Gunnoe, 2016). The majority of publications on academic functioning of IAPI children deals with those adopted before their second or third birthday—i.e., those who were in their adoptive families for three to four years before entering school. The literature on those IAPI children who entered the school system immediately after arriving in the US is minimal, although these children constitute about one-quarter of all international adoptees.

What are the criteria to judge the academic performance of IAPI students? In the majority of research reports, the following benchmarks are used:

• Academic grades reported by teachers.
• Results of academic achievement testing, either standardized tests or, in some cases, state-wide tests in reading and math.
• Number of referrals for special education services or placements.
• Actual special education placement according to educational classifications (the legally recognized educationally handicapping conditions in the US).
• Retention or delayed entry to school due to "readiness" issues.
• Teachers' and parents' surveys (opinions and judgments).

This is a rather diverse set of criteria. As a result, when the different points of reference are used, the obtained results are so different that they may confuse any reader. For example, in the meta-analysis of over 70 studies, Van IJzendoorn, Femmie Juffer, and Klein Poelhuis (2005) found that about 13% of IAPI children in North America were referred for special education placement compared to 5.5% among their non-adopted classmates. Completed roughly in the same decade (2000 to 2010), several other studies in North America and Western Europe indicated that by grade six, nearly 50% of international adoptees either had educational classifications (indication of academic handicapping conditions), were placed into special education programs, or had an average of two to four years of different special education services with their formal schooling (Meese, 2002, 2005; Tirella, Chan, & Miller, 2009; Werum, Cheng, & Browne, 2017; ref).

Other studies showed that adoptees were referred for special education at least twice as often as non-adoptees (Zill, 2015; Thomas, 2016), and those adopted after their fourth or fifth birthday are twice as likely to have learning problems that necessitate special education placement than those adopted before their second birthday (Van IJzendoorn & Juffer, 2006; Tirella et al., 2009). Teachers reported that IAPI children lag behind non-adopted classmates in academic achievements, as measured by academic tests, capacity to learn independently, participation in school-based academic activities, and productive peer engagement (LeMare, Vaughan, Watford, & Fernyhough, 2001; Judge, 2003; Meese, 2005; Welsh, Andres, Viana, Petrill, & Mathias, 2007; Welsh & Viana, 2012; Zill, 2015). Adopted children were more likely to repeat a grade or have learning disabilities that required enrollment in special classes (Ames,

Chisholm, Fisher, & Savoie, 1997; Hodges & Tizard, 1998; Dalen, 2001; Helder et al., 2016; White, 2017).

Claus and Baxter (1997) surveyed 206 adoptive families and found that 39% of adoptive families with children in elementary school reported learning problems ranging from speech and language, academic, and grapho-motor skills to peer interaction. Tirella et al. (2009) found that 83% of the children in their sample of 183 IAPI children ages 8 to 12 received special education services; specifically, 32% received occupational therapy, 52% had language disorders, 38% had problems with attention, and 36% had learning disabilities. Thirty-five percent had multiple neurodevelopmental diagnoses. Price (2000) also surveyed parents of 573 families that adopted 798 children. These children ranged in age from 1 year to 14 years at the time of adoption and lived with their adoptive parents on average about 8 years. In Price's survey, 25% of adoptive parents reported academic and language delays for their adopted children. Furthermore, Price found that the children were in their adoptive homes an average of 2.6 years before their academic and language issues became apparent to their parents when the children entered grades 1 through 5 in school. This is an important finding that confirms my empirical conclusion that a latent period takes place while cumulative cognitive deficit and academic difficulties surface in IAPI children. Another confirmation came from N. Zill (2015), who reported that the number of IAPI children who were classified as having special education needs grew with years of formal education, from 31% children in kindergarten to 54% children in 7th grade.

The important longitudinal perspectives were offered by the study of Romanian children adopted by Canadian parents. After about ten years in adoptive families, 29% of children exhibited significant attentional and cognitive/academic (math and reading comprehension) difficulties. These children were adopted before their second birthday, and in spite of tremendous rehabilitation/remediation efforts, still demonstrated poorer academic performance and lower ratings by teachers regarding schoolwork habits than family-raised children (Ames et al., 1997).

According to Western European reports, many of them being longitudinal studies, teachers perceive IAPI children as having more significant academic difficulties than their non-adopted classmates. Thus M. Dalen (2001) reported that her sample of 193 children adopted from Colombia and South Korea performed significantly lower than the matching group of Norwegian-born children. Most of the disparity was explained by poor language skills, a low ability to use the language at a higher cognitive level, and a high frequency of hyperactive behavior. Significant factors were the age at adoption and the country of origin, as Colombian children performed noticeably lower than their peers from South Korea.

In June of 2018, Adoption UK (the biggest Great Britain organization involved in international adoption[1]) published its report titled "Bridging the Gap: Giving Adopted Children an Equal Chance in School"[2]. The Adoption UK organization surveyed more than 2,000 adoptive parents and nearly 2,000 adopted young people to explore how effectively their social and emotional well-being was supported in school. The survey revealed the challenging daily reality of school life for adoptive families and their children in Great Britain. Thus IAPI children are more likely to be excluded; more likely to have social, emotional, and mental health difficulties; and more likely to leave school with no proper credentials. IAPI children achieve about half as well as their peers in statutory examinations and are 20 times more likely to be permanently excluded from school. With the link between social/emotional functioning and educational attainment so well documented, 79% of adopted young people agreed with the statement, "I feel confused and worried at school." Two-thirds of higher grades adolescents conveyed that they had been teased or bullied at school because they are adopted. Almost 70% of parents feel that their adopted children's progress in learning is affected by problems with their well-being in school and 60% of adoptive parents do not feel that their child has an equal chance at school.

The data presented in Zill's (2015) research show that adopted children in kindergarten and first grade display above-average levels of problem behavior, exhibit below-average levels of positive learning attitudes, and score below average on reading and math assessments, despite their advantageous adoptive family background. A new (2018) follow-up publication by Zill and Bradford was based on a longitudinal study conducted by the National Center for Education Statistics of a national sample of kindergarteners that included 160 adopted children. The results call into question a widely held assumption that larger investments of money and time in children can overcome the effects of early stress, deprivation, and genetic risk factors. The major finding indicated that academic problems of IAPI students multiply in middle school (see also N. Zill publication dated 2015, 2016). Thus by eighth grade, nearly half of adopted children have educational classifications of different learning-handicapped conditions. In the same sample, about 30% of students with a background in international adoption have received an out-of-school suspension by the end of that school year, compared to 10% of children living with biological parents. Adopted students performed significantly below average on reading, math, and science assessments on statewide tests. These figures were adjusted for differences across groups in students' average age, gender, and racial-ethnic composition; parent education; and family income levels. What is interesting, in Zill's new report there was no statistically significant difference between children adopted in infancy and those adopted later in life.

As children progress through the school system, the academic, social, and communication demands placed on them increase, and learning difficulties become more evident. Zill called this phenomenon "a puzzle of the Middle School (Zill, 2016)," and It is fully supported by clinical observations at the BGCenter: a substantial fraction of the adopted children who did not have diagnosed educational disabilities in the early grades were diagnosed with different educational incapacities in later grades.

It's likely that the rate of special needs services reflects the higher level of care and concern repeatedly evidenced by adoptive parents. However, there are two factors to bear in mind about these alarmingly high numbers presented earlier. First, most of the conditions with which adopted children are diagnosed are not severe intellectual impairments or clear-cut aggravated neurological disorders, but relatively less severe educational handicaps, such as "speech/language disorder," "emotional disturbance," "learning disability," or "attention-deficit hyperactivity disorder." Second, as Zill suggested, adoptive parents are especially sensitive to the health and well-being of their charges, and energetic in obtaining disability diagnoses and medical, psychiatric, and educational services for their adopted children. Adoptive parents typically were more informed about available services and more alert to potential problems than were non-adoptive parents and thus more likely to seek out such services and refer their children to them.

Causes of Poor Academic Functioning of IAPI Children

It would be practically important and instructive to find out why about one-third of international adoptees, presumably coming from the same damaging environment, have been doing well in school and do not need special education help. Based on the existing literature, we may distinguish the following factors that correlate with acceptable school performance:

- Age of adoption: generally, the younger the better, although adoption at a young age is not a guarantee of proper academic performance later. The decisive factor is that the time horizon for remediation is wider.
- Country of origin: statistically, children adopted from China and South Asia perform better academically than same age children from Russia, India, and Latin America. It is unclear why a vast majority of children adopted from South Korea are free from academic and cognitive problems. The fact is that the geography of adoption has relevance to proper academic performance (see Odenstad et al., 2008). It is likely that the quality of the orphanage system in the donating countries is a factor: this is particularly emphasized by some European researchers who came to the conclusion that the better the orphanage system, the easier it is for adopted children to

perform better in school later in life after adoption (Dalen, 2001; Tirella et al., 2009).

- Gender: across the board, adopted girls performed better than adopted boys in school (Lindblad, Dalen, Rasmussen, Vinnerljung, & Hjern, 2009).

The questions remained as to why so many IAPI children struggle so much in school in the Western school system in spite to the fact that adoptive parents and school personnel apply extraordinary resources, time, and patience educating IAPI children. In the research literature, there are plenty of attempts to explain this phenomenon, and these explanations do have points, to different degrees. Thus a genetic endowment theory, supported by Miller (2005), Zill (2015, 2016) and a number of other researchers appears relevant. The individuals adopting internationally cannot choose or control the genetic bequest of the children they adopt; most children available for adoption are likely to have a less favorable intellectual/academic accomplishment than their adoptive parents. No matter how much intellectual stimulation and encouragement the parents provide, they may not be able to overcome the limitations of the child's genetic heritage.

The review of research literature combined with our clinical experience allows us to establish subjective and objective factors that negatively affect the school performance of IAPI children. The subjective (related to children) factors are

- language transition upon a generally weak language foundation and an abrupt attrition of the first language,
- limited or complete lack of academic readiness,
- CCD in "older" adoptees (see Chapter 5),
- maladaptive behaviors instilled by trauma and institutional life, and
- lack of motivation to achieve academically due to the negative self-perception.

All these factors are the consequences of extreme educational neglect combined with repetitive stressful events that affect all domains of an IAPI child's life, including the leading activity: learning in school. Trauma affects learning through a number of venues. Thus an orphanage background shapes behavior through its impact on a child's aspirations, sense of efficacy, and personal standards of achievements. As students, IAPI children have a fear of failure due to past experiences. Some of them can be capable of a task at hand, but they believe that they cannot learn as a result of previous demoralizing experiences or self-imposed mind-sets. If they doubt their academic ability, chances are they envision low grades before they even complete an assignment or take a test, creating an effect on goal setting: these children tend to set lower goals for themselves and have little incentive to persevere in the face of difficulty. Many of the difficulties IAPI students encounter in school are closely connected to beliefs they hold about themselves and their place in the world (see Chapter 3 for the "internal working model" in IAPI children).

Among subjective factors, self-perception as "incapable," a fear of school failure, and school-related anxiety constitute significant obstacles for successful learning. It was our clinical experience, based on years of communicating with schoolteachers and adoptive parents, that due to general incompetence and low self-confidence, IAPI children may lack the ability to successfully join in group activities and do not experience the feelings of competency that results from those endeavors. The inability to work cooperatively in groups can significantly impact school functioning given the social nature of learning in the classroom.

The objective factors (related to school as an institution) for school difficulties of IAPI children include

- the inability of our school system to recognize and address unique educational needs of IAPI students,
- a lack of remedial methodologies for IAPI children in our schools, and
- inappropriate school placement and the issue of remediation versus mainstream education;

These factors mean no less than the continuation of traumatic experiences in IAPI children; this is "de facto" educational neglect and further traumatization of IAPI children in our school systems. Let us consider the objective factors in more detail, starting with such concepts as academic readiness and proper school placement for IAPI children.

Academic Readiness in the Context of International Adoption

School "readiness" is a structured set of competencies relevant to societal expectations for a certain chronological age. Readiness is always a continuum (a range) of competencies that may be roughly described as "deficient," "below average," "average," or "above average" in relation to the majority of a child's peers (Winsler & Carlton, 1999). When readiness is considered, it is mostly about school entry by a young child. However, in the context of international adoption, readiness really needs to be considered for all age levels, as the IAPI children are adopted from all age groups, from 3 months through 17 years. Their academic readiness is very multifaceted.

The very concept of readiness is controversial, as well as ways of defining it (Lewitt & Baker, 1995). Does it relate to the child's age, health, skills, social/emotional maturity, or the results of special tests? According to the apple-or-coin test used in the Middle Ages, children were to start school when they were mature enough for delayed gratification and had the abstract reasoning involved in choosing money over a fruit. Since the Middle Ages, not much progress has been made in this domain: there are no selection criteria, universal tests, or even commonly agreed upon sets of behaviors that allow parents and professionals to decide whether a child is ready for formal schooling. Legally, the only requirement for academic placement in the US is the chronological age of the child; thus, children must be 5 years old by September 1 (or January 1 in some states) for kindergarten entrance, 6 for first grade, 7 for second grade, 8 for third grade, and so on.

The concept of academic readiness is inherently controversial because children learn and develop at a different pace. For example, clear articulation may be achieved by some children by the age of 4, and others only by the age of 8, while the majority will speak clearly by age of 6. All of this is still considered "normal" by most speech pathologists (Bernthal, Bankson, & Flipsen, 2013). The same goes for many self-help skills, decoding of printed words, following multiple directions, etc. No wonder we see children with wide variations in their school-related skills in typical kindergarten through third grade classes.

The Components of Academic Readiness

There are four intertwined but still distinct factors playing a role in the academic readiness of a child: 1) language as a means of learning and mediator of literacy skills, 2) cognitive ability to learn specific skills and knowledge, 3) academic or pre-academic skills and knowledge, and 4) social and emotional competence to function in school as an institution and to participate in shared activities with others. These four factors of school readiness, being powerful inhibitors or facilitators of learning, do not always develop in harmony: a child may be ready cognitively or language-wise but be very immature socially, or vice versa. The vast majority of school-age international adoptees are not prepared for the school experience in Western schools upon arrival in all the aforementioned domains of school readiness.

I wrote about the language issues in IAPI children in Chapter 4, and it is clear that in this domain, the readiness for school functioning for all ages is way below the age expectations compared to their classmates. Remediation in cognitive language deficit should go hand in hand with the process of second-language acquisition in international adoptees. Due to the speech (articulation, fluency, etc.) and language deficits and delays, many international adoptees have been found eligible for speech and language services in public schools; in fact, this is the remedial educational service most frequently offered to them (see Chapter 4).

Social skills and the ability to participate in shared activities are important indicators of readiness. The capacity to initiate, respond to, and maintain social interaction is a must in school due to the very nature of the school environment. With its emphasis on collaboration, teamwork, and project-based activity, school presents a high demand on a child's social skills. In addition, a teacher-pupil interaction comes into play: social skills are needed to interact with an adult in a teaching position. Self-regulation becomes a major part of social/emotional competency: this is the basic requirement for functioning in school and an indication of the child's emotional and social maturity. Self-regulation is needed for what is called "goal-directed behavior" socially as well academically. As presented in Chapter 6, emotional vulnerability in international adoptees in the school context makes them less able to tolerate stress as expected for their age, less capable of self-regulating their goal-directed behavior, and less self-sufficient in overcoming the emotional strain while competing in school.

Cognitive competence in children ready for formal education in school includes fundamental abilities and processes, such as classification, pattern detection, comparison, association, concept formation, acknowledging similarities and differences, identifying basic solutions of visual puzzles, and increasing attention and focus to challenging tasks. These capacities could be tested through standardized psychological tests. As it was explained in Chapter 5, many basic cognitive skills in typically developing child are formed in their preschool years through direct and mediated learning. These cognitive competencies are further developing during school-based learning and formed the base for math, writing, and reading proficiencies. However, in many school-age IAPI children, this foundation has not been formed due to educational neglect and deprivation in their preschool and elementary school years, and it is much more difficult for them to master literacy skills. Limited cognitive readiness, as described in Chapter 5, affects the overall school readiness.

Academic and pre-academic skills, as a component of school readiness, are usually measured by a wide range of standardized educational tests, with all their possibilities and limitations in terms of psychometric properties and practical utility. In my opinion, these tests are grossly inappropriate for IAPI children: by default, children with an institutional background have a huge disadvantage compared to their counterparts living in middle-class birth families. Among other things, they do not have the same cultural experiences as their classmates: the use of home computers; visits to parks, museums, and theaters; attending preschool programs; availability of literature and educational reading materials; or interactions with educated, literate, and well-spoken, emotionally involved adults. IAPI children lack these mutually satisfying social interactions. As the result, they are delayed in regard to many pre-academic and academic skills and accomplishments. We do know that their specific knowledge base is weaker and different from the one acquired by their peers in

American schools. Our diagnostic questions should be their amenability to academic instruction and guidance, their cognitive modifiability, their responsiveness to an adult's mediation and intervention. That is what we need to know for effective remediation, and that is the ultimate goal of educational assessment.

At BGCenter, when assessing newly arrived preschool and school-age IAPI children in their native languages, we have been using the Application of Cognitive Functions Scale (ACFS—authors are Carol Lidz and Ruthanne Jepsen[3]). Although we basically followed the procedure presented by Lidz[4] (Haywood & Lidz, 2007), we used this procedure in our own adaptation, at time all six scales and at other times only four scales. Each activity was presented in a "dynamic format": first we ask the child to engage in the pre-academic or academic activities without adult assistance, to demonstrate the child's independent functioning. The intervention segment offers standard assistance that emphasizes the strategies and type of processing that is involved in successful completion of the activity (Lidz & Gindis, 2003). We mostly used the ACFS diagnostically or for individual exploration of the child's functioning in the areas tapped by the activities. I consider dynamic assessment (in a format presented by Lidz, 2003; Haywood & Lidz, 2007) as a viable alternative to standardized academic tests in initial screening and testing of IAPI children upon arrival.

Current options for the IAPI children who are "not ready" for the age-appropriate school experience, in their parents' and teachers' opinion, include delayed entry to kindergarten or first grade, retention for another year in the same grade, lower-grade attendance, enrollment into an "inclusion" or "transitional" class, or special education placement.

In terms of educational placement, parents and teachers have to take IAPI children's actual developmental status and level of functioning as a reference point and not just their chronological age. Emotional, cognitive, and behavioral immaturity is the "trademark" of post-institutionalized children. A mismatch between the child's learning capacity and academic placement is a recipe for a traumatic school experience. Unfortunately, school personnel often do not know how to address the specificity of international adoptees, "how to fit these square pegs into the round holes of existing special ed. programs" as one parent said. With international adoptees, remedial efforts should be as diversified as the causes of their educational difficulties.

The Concept of Bidirectionality in Academic Placement of IAPI Children

The major pitfall of the current school readiness practices in relation to IAPI children is rooted in the belief that readiness is totally within the child, and he or she is required to demonstrate readiness before entering the school system or a specific grade. When the parents and educational professionals decide that the readiness resides solely in the child's properties, and if age-appropriate placement is clearly unsuitable, they have to restrict themselves to the three options mentioned earlier: delayed entry (for preschoolers), retention, or below the age-appropriate grade placement.

There is another perspective on the issue of school readiness, discussed in Winsler and Carlton (1999) and Berk and Winsler (1995) publications. It is called the "bidirectional approach," implying that readiness resides in the child-school interconnectedness. Within the bidirectional approach, a child and a school are considered an interconnected entity adjusted to each other. Let us consider the following child- and school-referenced criteria for such interconnectedness in the context of IAPI child's readiness.

Child-referenced criteria may include chronological age, which is an important, but not decisive factor; general health; language development; social skills and ability to participate in shared activity; self-regulation; age-appropriate cognitive competence; and specific school-related academic or pre-academic skills.

School-referenced criteria may include experience with international adoptees, willingness of the administration and teachers to modify their standard curriculum and test requirements, a schedule to accommodate an IAPI child's unique needs, quality of the ESL program, support services within regular education, availability of remedial programs outside of special education, and the availability of special education programs and services.

Scaffolded experiences within the school setting allow IAPI children to form practical readiness for mainstream education. A child does not merely grow into readiness, but must be exposed to situations and be carefully assisted by others to develop the necessary skills and ways of functioning. The bidirectional model is closely connected with the concepts of "zone of proximal development" and "scaffolding," as discussed in Chapter 3 of this book. Working with an IAPI child who is not ready for age-appropriate instruction, and using the scaffolding methodology, the teacher is to moderate an assignment's difficulty to keep it at a properly challenging level for the child. As explained by Haywood and Lidz (2007), the teacher is to monitor the amount of assistance provided to the child, gradually withdrawing the amount of joint/shared activity as soon as the child's competence increases. The teacher is to apply leading questions (and other problem-solving strategies) to assist the child with the task. As the metaphor "scaffolding" suggests, the overall goal of this teaching/learning approach is to gradually develop a child's competence while carefully and gradually removing the support (scaffolding). An example of scaffolding teaching/learning procedure with an IAPI child can be found in Gindis and Karpov's publication (2000).

Damaging Misconception About IAPI Children in School

The promotion of the bidirectional approach in developing the academic readiness of IAPI children requires that school personnel be informed about many misconceptions about these children. Here are just a few major notions that are common for public and school personnel but have no basis:

- IAPI children are considered to be similar to children from recently immigrated families and therefore should be educated the same way, placed academically according to their chronological age, and taught ESL the same way. Parents would be generally advised to "wait and see" how their children adjust to the new social/cultural and school environment.
- IAPI children are seen by the school personnel as "bilingual." This leads to many unfortunate consequences in terms of remediation when ESL instructional services are considered as the means, often the only one, of addressing IAPI children with language and learning issues. School staff members continue to believe that IAPI children "keep" their languages and fail to consider that an abrupt language loss and its cognitive and academic consequences lead to an educational handicapping condition in some children.
- Among school personnel, there is a belief that no testing should be done before the children learn English. This is in direct contradiction to the major educational law, IDEA-2004, that clearly stated that tests and other evaluation materials used to assess a child are to be provided and administered in the child's native language (IDEA 34 CFR 300.532(a)(ii[5]).
- Many school teachers and administrators think, that both academic and behavioral, are solely due to the children's institutional background and no learning or other disability exists, but rather just consequences from being raised in an orphanage. Loving families, good nutrition, and consistent schooling are all these children need for recovery.
- School teachers assume that international adoptees may not be eligible for special education services because of the language and cultural issues involved.
- School personnel believes, that school age IAPI children should continue their education from the grade level they were in their native countries. This specific misconception is particularly damaging, because it leads to a grossly inappropriate school placement. The grade placement in the country of origin should not serve as a base for the school placement in the US/Canada educational systems. It is likely that adopted children have significant gaps and breaches in their academic knowledge base that are assumed to be present and adequate in a child of their age

who was raised in a birth family. No significant transfer of academic skills from the native language curriculum to American curriculum should be expected. In my clinical experience, providing psychoeducational testing of internationally adopted children from Eastern Europe and the Russian Federation in particular, I found that too many of the school-aged children perform from 2 to 4 grades below their claimed grade placement in Russia when tested against the standard Russian curriculum. Several years of deprivation and educational neglect result in the majority of IA children having an astonishing lack of age-appropriate skills and the ability to regulate their internal psychological processes. These children are very much in need of remediation along with education, and it is often a big mistake to decide on their school placement based on the placement in the country of origin.

Such assumptions are damaging for internationally adopted post-institutionalized children, depriving them of needed help and support in education. School personnel view them through the unavoidable cultural lenses. What the pedagogical staff members see when a child is brought to the school for the first time are either one or two well-educated, predominantly middle-class parents who present to them a good-looking, nicely dressed child. In the eyes of teachers, there is no difference between this newcomer and the family-raised children from the same socioeconomic strata; they do not realize that the child often lacks fundamental pieces of normal development that will be reflected in academic problems later on. In most cases, this a deeply traumatized child, and the consequences will affect the learning process and school-based socialization. All children who fall behind deserve immediate intervention, but for IAPI children, it's crucial: only a few of them can catch up on their own. For most of them, early intervention is the only thing that will keep them moving along; without such scaffold, they are doomed to failure.

Academic Remediation and Special Education Options for IAPI Children

The academic "profile" of many IAPI children (particular those adopted at school-age—after their fifth birthday) includes signs of learning impediments: they display constant forgetting of learned material and the inability to transfer knowledge and skills from one situation to another; lack of age-expected learning strategies; cognitive language deficiency, often concurrent with age-appropriate social "everyday" language; immature self-regulation of behavior, resulting in poor concentration and limited attention span; and diminished intrinsic motivation for learning or achieving in learning activities. The psychological issues (described in Chapter 5) behind these observable patterns of learning behavior often predefine academic failure, reinforcing low self-esteem, lack of interest in studying, and constant frustration associated with learning efforts.

When a child has missed certain stages of normal development and has never learned the skills and concepts necessary for successful schooling, the educational matter this child is taught simply does not have any structural cognitive support upon which to be understood, remembered, and used. As presented in Chapter 5, the psychological roots of many learning problems for IAPI children are due to a lack of a viable foundation to productively develop more complex cognitive skills and processes. For many IAPI children adopted at school-age, academic placement below chronological age in combination with remedial programming (in or outside of special education) is the right way to go: we have to restore the foundations before proceeding to teach more advanced academic skills to reverse damage done to their learning capacity in the past.

In other words, many, if not the majority of IAPI children, need remediation before being a part of the mainstream education classroom. The notion of "remediation" means "to rectify, improve or remedy something." Remedial education is designed to scaffold a student who lacks basic learning skills and knowledge to achieve expected competencies for continuation in the mainstream educational process. Both students with and without educational disability may benefit from remedial education.

Remedial programs are not the same as special education programs. Remedial programs are designed to restore the basis for learning more advanced academic skills and knowledge in children who may not have an identifiable learning disability, while special education is designed to meet the needs of students with educational disabilities. However, there are three attributes that are common for remedial and special education programs: 1) they require specialized instructions that are different from the mainstream teaching, 2) they take place (in most cases, but not always) outside of a regular classroom, and 3) they are taught by specially trained teachers.

Some IAPI children may not benefit from remedial programs and should be evaluated for the presence of educational handicapping conditions and the need for more specialized instruction or a more individualized setting. An effective remedial program is expected to use research-based specialized teaching methods; be consistent and systematic; be presented at an appropriate individualized pace, include pre-teaching, repetitions, and practices; and be taught in a small group or individually.

There is a rather complicated relationship between academic readiness, remedial services, and special education eligibility. In school practice, a lack of readiness for a certain grade level can be used for the denial of remediation and special education services: it is assumed that just waiting a year before entering kindergarten or retaining the child in the same grade is sufficient for recovery. This is grossly inappropriate for IAPI children.

Academic remediation of IAPI children should take place on two levels: at school and at home. In school, remedial instruction can be in or outside of special education. In general, remedial methodologies in different disciplines (e.g., literacy, speech, and language, occupational therapy) developed for the general population may be applicable for IAPI children with some modifications, if needed. There is a wide range of such methodologies presented in a number of publications (Lidz, 2003; Gindis, 2006; Welsh et al., 2007; Haywood & Lidz, 2007). Federal law (IDEA-2004) strongly supports remediation in general education settings (34 CFR Sec. 300.116(e)).

To qualify for special education, a child must have an educational handicapping condition recognized by IDEA-2004. The school's legal obligations to children with any of the recognized educational handicaps is to be spelled out in the child's Individual Educational Plan (IEP), which contains educational classification (a description of educational needs for which a child must receive remedial help in school), statements about educational needs, goals of remediation and means of accountability in reaching goals, teaching remedial methodologies, classroom accommodations, and test-taking modifications.

The IEP is to be based on a comprehensive and focused assessment of an IAPI child's needs (see Addendum 2: Samples of 1) Initial Bilingual Psychoeducational Screening and 2) Comprehensive Neuropsychological and Educational Assessment). Any evaluation of an IAPI child referred due to learning problems should answer the following questions:

- What are the child's educational needs?
- Does the child qualify for educational classification?
- What is the most appropriate educational placement?
- What supportive and remedial help does the child need?
- What are the goals of remediation?
- What are the methods of remediation?
- How should progress be measured?

As for home remediation of cognitive and language issues, at this time, there is only one remedial cognitive and language remedial methodology developed specifically for IAPI children: SmartStart (Lidz & Gindis, 2006). This methodology considers the specificity of international adoptees, does not require special skills or training from the adoptive parents, promotes attachment and bonding, is a family affair (not a school-like activity because the parents should not be second-shift teachers), complements school-based remediation, and addresses emotional needs along with cognitive issues.

One of the lessons learned within the 30 years of international adoption on a wide scale is that many, likely the majority of IAPI children, need remediation (remedial instructions), some (significant minority that has educational handicapping conditions) need special education services, and some need special education placement and services temporarily or for the whole length of their schooling. However, intensive, focused research in this area is urgently needed to verify the effectiveness of existing remedial and special education methodologies in relation to IAPI children and guide our practical recommendations. In order to make remedial treatments more effective, the uniqueness of international adoptees should be taken into consideration, and existing methods should be appropriately modified and adjusted to meet the challenges presented by IAPI children.

I started this book with a clinical case description that I titled "Alex—An Enigmatic Source of Strength." I would like to conclude with the clinical case description where the source of success is known and quite evident.

Clinical Case: Diana—The Evident Source of Strength

I read this letter from Nicole with a feeling of wonder that had unfolded before my eyes over the last 14 years:

> *Diana is going to Tokyo in March with her photography professor and four other photography students for a workshop. She is the little engine that never gives up. She will be graduating college this December! Who would have thought it would ever happen? She is applying to a very high-end fine arts photography studio in our town that is opening in January to be a photography assistant. She already met the owner and showed him her portfolio. It would be great, but it is not yet confirmed. She is working this summer as an arts and crafts counselor at a children's camp.*

In my office 14 years ago, I saw a fragile and scared 7-year-old girl with all of the classical signs of FASD: weight, height, and head circumference below the third percentile for her age and typical facial features, such as slanted eyes, no philtrum (the vertical indentation in the middle area of the upper lip), thin upper lip, and other typical facial characteristics of FASD. Her biological mother was designated as an "alcohol abuser" in the legal adoption documents. Diana spent the four years before adoption in a small orphanage located in a remote rural area and never attended school. Her psychological examination upon arrival showed significant delays and impairments of her higher psychological functions (memory, language, attention, etc.) with cognitive functioning within the Low Average to Borderline range.

Her adoptive mother, Nicole, a middle-aged single parent and an accomplished lawyer, looked at me with a mix of hope and anxiety: "What does the future hold for us?" I briefly explained the psychological, educational, and social consequences of intrauterine exposure to alcohol, information that seemed to be new to Nicole. I said that if she wanted to see her newly adopted daughter functioning close to her age expectations at the age of 21, she must invest enormous amounts of effort, time, and money into Diana's rehabilitation and remediation because of Diana's significant neurologically based limitations. College? Likely not. Nicole was understandably upset with my verdict, but in the waiting room, she suddenly hugged Diana and kissed her profusely. She turned to me and said, "Please write the most comprehensive remedial program for my daughter."

"I can write the 'ideal' program, but I doubt that the school will be able to implement it; the school is looking for 'the most appropriate,' not 'the optimal' program."

"Don't worry. They will do all that is necessary" replied Nicole with a suddenly resolute tone of voice.

From day one, Nicole took a methodical, well-thought-out, and persistent approach to Diana's remediation and physical and emotional restoration. It was almost a business plan: with goals, methods, responsibilities of executors, and deadlines. One may skeptically make a face reading this, but it worked! She called it a "Road Map to Recovery" and constantly reviewed and modified it. In setting her goals, Nicole was realistic, but still optimistic. She wanted to be proactive rather than reactive to Diana's needs. It was amazing how skillful Nicole was in creating an expert team to support and guide her road map. In addition to a psychologist, at different times, the team included a speech pathologist, an educational attorney (one of the best I've ever met), a physician (specializing in international adoption medicine and a known expert on FASD), an occupational therapist, a physical therapist, psychotherapists, and counselors, and several tutors in different subjects. All these specialists were available on an as-needed basis, and Nicole was as effective a manager of this group as one can imagine (how she was able to combine this with a ten-hour day in her law firm is beyond me, but she managed). It was a substantial financial investment as well: expertise costs! However, her money was wisely invested and resulted in psychological and mental health gains that could not be measured in numbers.

Diana's school district in an affluent Boston suburb enthusiastically accepted my comprehensive remedial plan—a rather rare case in my experience. Diana was placed in a small, self-contained class designed for children with language impairments and learning disabilities. She received the educational services and support, and as an extra perk, she had a one-on-one paraprofessional for her first year in school. Still, the beginning was very difficult, and Diana went through constant struggles and had trouble keeping up with even the modified and individualized school program. Frequent frustrations, tears, and withdrawals showed her emotional instability. Her first two years in a public school were neither happy nor productive. Nicole decided that public school wasn't giving her daughter enough.

Not too far from their home was one of the best private special education schools with an outstanding reputation. It was one of a few private special education schools organized according to the classic British system of education, where, in addition to small class instructions, every child had an adult mentor for one-on-one instruction. It was a very expensive school. Nicole studied the place relentlessly, interviewed parents and staff, and then decided, "This is it."

"The school district is going to cover her tuition costs," Nicole decided. "I have lived here all my life and have paid many thousands in school taxes. Let them pick up the tab this time." She formed a new team of experts: a lawyer, a medical doctor, and a speech pathologist. I participated as a psychologist. With her systematic approach and excellent organization skills, Nicole was able to gain the upper hand in her negotiations and received the district's commitment to pay for Diana's special education at a private institution as the girl had unique educational needs, unmet by the school district. The initial commitment covered three years and was later extended until middle school.

Diana did well in her new school both academically and emotionally, but not without pitfalls. Some of the problems were "typical adolescent stuff" and Diana just took her share. One of the many characteristics of FASD is that these children are easily influenced by others: the underlying impairment of their frontal lobes affects high-order reasoning and executive functions, and impedes independent judgment, making it difficult to anticipate consequences. The lack of understanding of ownership, belongings, lending versus giving, taking versus borrowing are all typical misjudgments in individuals with FASD; it's a cognitive inability rather than a moral flaw.

Having weak inner "stoppers," Diana occasionally violated school rules and regulations, and she faced disciplinary actions, including suspension. Every day brought new challenges, and nothing came easily. The school used an effective and highly structured multisensory remedial program for reading with disabled students. By the ninth grade, Diana reached the sixth-grade level in reading and writing, but her math skills—the hardest subject for students with FASD—stayed at a fourth-grade level.

Diana was not conventionally pretty, athletic, or smart, and had nothing to distinguish her among her peers. To raise her daughter's self-esteem, Nicole encouraged Diana to search for a channel in which she could prove herself, and soon they found it.

While struggling academically and socially, Diana was very perceptive and imaginative. Art became her breath of fresh air, an outlet to escape reality. A special tutor was invited to develop Diana's drawing skills and painting techniques. She did still life, went out for plain-air painting on weekends, and never parted with her sketchpad. In her church, Diana tutored young children to draw and do photography. When she got seriously interested in photography, Nicole bought every possible piece of equipment from a good camera and lenses to flash and tripods to support her daughter's new undertaking.

Diana stood out from her peers in visual arts achievements, and Nicole realized that it was the right direction to focus their efforts on. She never reproached Diana for poor grades, but praised her for the achievements in arts, in which the girl excelled, including participating in local exhibitions and getting praises and honorable mentions. The girl's portfolio and self-esteem were improving along with her mother's excitement over her daughter's rehabilitation. Nicole started looking for another school.

In a neighboring state, there was a so-called magnet school (arts-oriented charter high school)—a public education collaborative project that functioned as an extension of the local school districts. This small school was specifically designed for students with developmental and social deficiencies who were advanced creatively; they embraced dancers, musicians, and those taking up fine art like Diana.

Initially, this art school rejected Diana's application. The art portfolio received the highest marks, but the academic grades were below the passing threshold, particularly math: a person who calculated no higher than the fourth-grade level could not be a high school student. Not being deterred, Nicole had every member of her support team (a lawyer, a physician, and a psychologist) write letters to the state educational authorities. Nicole involved an influential group of National Organization of Fetal Alcohol Syndrome to put pressure not on the school—the scale was way too small for them—but on the State Educational Department, which in turn sent their directives to the school administrators. Finally, Nicole obtained an appointment with the state educational commissioner and convinced him to accept Diana, even with delayed academic skills. The school resorted to one final excuse: "You live outside our state; we have no buses to come and pick up your daughter from so far away." Nicole had rented an apartment near the school and began commuting to Boston herself—two hours one-way every day.

As Diana continued to pursue art, she made a sudden leap in her academics. She did so well that she was able to pass a GED exam, which meant that she would graduate with a regular high school diploma, not a special education one. She barely had a passing grade in math, but her SAT results, although far from spectacular, proved high enough to secure college acceptance.

Diana applied to several colleges, all art related, and Nicole chose a small suburban school in upstate New York, about a five-hour drive from their home in Massachusetts. Let us go back to the letter I cited in the beginning of this story:

> *This past semester was extremely difficult with upper divisional courses in Chinese Philosophy and Western Literature. Beyond hard. I got my sister who is a retired math teacher to read the books and tutor Diana by verbally, discussing with her concepts and ideas*

and arguments. Then they created bulleted worksheets, and Diana wrote sample essays, as the tests were all essay based. They worked extremely hard many hours a week, and Diana got a B and a C in those courses! This is an amazing feat and accomplishment for Diana! I am beyond proud of her!

Let's put this into perspective. If someone told me when I had just met Diana that she would go to a college, I would have sworn that it was impossible. Even as late as her high school sophomore year, the claim would have remained a low-percentage gamble, but both Diana and her mother proved me wrong with their persistence and dedication.

An amazing aspect of human development is that this success even affected Diana's physical appearance. She passed the ugly duckling stage and turned into a pretty young adult. She is still petite, but her face transformed, softening the signs of her disorder. She is always nicely dressed and wears sophisticated makeup. Diana's church selected her to be a part of the youth delegation to meet with the Pope in Rome. Nicole decided to go with her, and a picture from the stairs of St. Peter's Cathedral stays on the shelf in my office: a nice-looking young lady in fashionable glasses and a bright scarf, and behind her is her mom, with such happiness radiating from her face that no explanation is needed. The very fact that this girl with such a heavy neurological disability has overcome the odds and achieved the unthinkable is short of a miracle.

In 2011, I began a program called "FASD in School" with the goal of creating a network of specialists who would help students afflicted with FASD to receive everything necessary from the school district during their studies. Diana created the poster for the program (a mother polar bear and two cubs) which is still on our website: www.bgcenter.com/BGCenterServices/FASDinSchoolProject.htm.

Diana's example shows how vision, entrepreneurial skills, and, let's not overlook it, money turned a nearly hopeless child into a successful contributing member of society. It turned out that the battle against organic deficiency is not always a totally lost cause: inborn talent that is identified and supported early on may have the upper hand—exactly what happened with Diana.

Let me finish with one more excerpt from Nicole's letter:

My take away message is twofold: FASD kids can do the impossible if they are driven to succeed and have it as their goal, and, secondly, there must be a parent behind them who can obtain professional support services and direct the learning process through the institutions on their behalf. This was no journey for the faint of heart, and there was no template on how to do it, and it continues. My message for adoptive parents is this: Always be vigilant and aware of even the slightest behavioral changes and signs of your adopted child, no matter how much work you and your child may have done on the road to success, and seek help quickly! I have a bag of professional resources to go to at any time! I call it watching for the other shoe to drop! Or measured optimism. These kids are riding a bike with training wheels, and until they learn to ride without them, there are always challenges.

Notes

1. www.adoptionuk.org/
2. www.basw.co.uk/system/files/resources/bridging-the-gap.pdf
3. www.bgcenter.com/ACFS.htm
4. https://ir.vanderbilt.edu/handle/1803/4658?show=full
5. www.law.cornell.edu/cfr/text/34/300.304

References

Ames, E., Chisholm, K., Fisher, L., & Savoie, L. (1997). Problems reported by parents of Romanian orphans adopted to British Columbia. *International Journal of Behavioral Development, 20*(1), 77–82.

Beckett, C., Castle, J., Rutter, M., & Sonuga-Barke, E. J. (2010). Institutional deprivation, specific cognitive functions, and scholastic achievement: English and Romanian Adoptee (ERA) study findings. *Monographs of the Society for Research in Child Development, 75*, 125–142.

Berk, L. E., & Winsler, A. (1995). *Scaffolding children's learning: Vygotsky and early childhood education.* Washington, DC: National Association for the Education of Young Children.

Bernthal, J., Bankson, N. W., & Flipsen, P., Jr. (2013). *Articulation and phonological disorders.* New York, NY: Pearson.

Clauss, D., & Baxter, S. (1997). *Post adoption survey of Russian and Eastern European children.* Belen, NM: Rainbow House International.

Dalen, M. (2001). School performances among internationally adopted children in Norway. *Adoption Quarterly, 5*(2), 39–58.

Dole, K. (2005). Education and internationally adopted children: Working collaboratively with schools. *Pediatric Clinic of North America, 52*(5), 1445–1461.

Gindis, B. (1998). Navigating uncharted waters: School psychologists working with internationally adopted post-institutionalized children. *NASP Communiqué*, Part I: 27(1), 6–9; Part II: 27(2), 20–23.

Gindis, B. (2006). Cognitive, language, and educational issues of children adopted from overseas orphanages. *Journal of Cognitive Education and Psychology, 4*(3), 290–315.

Gindis, B., & Karpov, Y. V. (2000). Dynamic assessment of the level of internalization of elementary school children's problem-solving activity. In C. S. Lidz & J. G. Elliott (Eds.), *Dynamic assessment: Prevailing models and applications* (pp. 133–154). Amsterdam: Elsevier Science.

Haywood, H. C., & Lidz, C. (2007). *Dynamic assessment in practice: Clinical and educational applications.* Cambridge: Cambridge University Press.

Helder, E., Mulder, E., & Linder Gunnoe, M. (2016). A longitudinal investigation of children internationally adopted at school age. *Child Neuropsychology: Journal on Normal and Abnormal Development in Childhood and Adolescence, 22*(1), 39–64.

Hodges, J., & Tizard, B. (1998). The effect of early institutional rearing on the development of eight-year-old children. *Journal of Child Psychology & Psychiatry, 29*(1), 99–118.

Judge, S. (2003). Developmental recovery and deficit in children adopted from Eastern European Orphanages. *Child Psychiatry and Human Development, 34*, 49–62.

LeMare, L., Vaughan, K., Watford, L., & Fernyhough, L. (2001). *Intellectual and academic performance of Romanian orphans 10 years after being adopted to Canada.* Paper presented at the biennial meeting of the Society for Research in Child Development, Minneapolis, MN.

Lewitt, E. M., & Baker, L. S. (1995). School readiness. *Critical Issues for Children and Youths, 5*, 128–139.

Lidz, C. (2003). *Early childhood assessment.* Hoboken, NJ: John Wiley & Sons.

Lidz, C., & Gindis, B. (2003). Dynamic assessment of the evolving cognitive functions in children chapter 10. In A. Kozulin, B. Gindis, V. Ageyev, & S. Miller (Eds.), *Vygotsky educational theory in cultural context* (pp. 99–119). New York: Cambridge University Press.

Lidz, C., & Gindis, B. (2006). Take charge: Home-based cognitive and language remediation for internationally adopted children. *Adoption Today, 8*(4), 52–63.

Lindblad, F., Dalen, M., Rasmussen, F., Vinnerljung, B., & Hjern, A. (2009). School performance of international adoptees better than expected from cognitive test results. *European Child & Adolescent Psychiatry, 18*(5), 301–318.

Meese, R. L. (2002). *Children of intercountry adoptions in school: A primer for parents and professionals.* Westport, CT: Bergin & Garvey.

Meese, R. L. (2005). A few new children: Post-institutionalized children of intercountry adoption. *Journal of Special Education, 39*(3), 157–167.

Miller, L. (2005). *The handbook of international adoption medicine: A guide for physicians, parents, and provides.* New York: Oxford University Press.

Odenstad, A., Hjern, A., Lindblad, F., Rasmussen, F., Vinnerljung, B., & Dalen, M. (2008). Does age at adoption and geographic origin matter? A national cohort study of cognitive test performance in adult inter-country adoptees. *Psychological Medicine, 38*, 1803–1814.

Price, P. (2000). FRUA's health and development survey. *The Family Focus, 6*(3), 1–3.

Thomas, K. (2016). Adoption, foreign-born status, and children's progress in school. *Journal of Marriage and Family, 78*(1), 75–90.

Tirella, L., Chan, W., & Miller, L. (2009). Educational outcomes of children adopted from Eastern Europe, now ages 8–12. *Journal of Research in Childhood Education, 20*(4), 245–254.

Van IJzendoorn, M. H., Femmie Juffer, F., & Klein Poelhuis, C. (2005). Adoption and cognitive development: A meta-analytic comparison of adopted and nonadopted children's IQ and school performance. *Psychological Bulletin, 131*(2), 301–316.

Van IJzendoorn, M. H., & Juffer, F. (2006). Adoption as intervention: Meta-analytic evidence for massive catch-up and plasticity in physical, socio-emotional and cognitive development: The Emanuel Miller Memorial Lecture 2006. *Journal of Child Psychology and Psychiatry, 47*, 1128–1245.

Welsh, J., Andres, G., Viana, A., Petrill, S., & Mathias, M. (2007). Interventions for internationally adopted children and families: A review of the literature. *Child and Adolescent Social Work Journal, 24*, 285–311.

Welsh, J., & Viana, A. (2012). Developmental outcomes of internationally adopted children. *Adoption Quarterly, 15*(4), 241–264.

White, R. (2017). *Adoption UK's schools & exclusions report.* Banbury: Adoption, UK.

Winsler, A., & Carlton, M. (1999). School readiness: The need for a paradigm shift. *School Psychology Review, 28*(3), 338–352.

Zill, N. (2015). The paradox of adoption. *Publication of the Institute for Family Studies.* Retrieved July 19, 2018, from https://ifstudies.org/blog/the-paradox-of-adoption

Zill, N. (2016). How adopted children fare in middle school. *Publication of the Institute of Family Studies.* Retrieved from https://ifstudies.org/blog/how-adopted-children-fare-in-middle-school

Zill, N., & Bradford, W. (2018). The adoptive difference: New evidence on how adopted children perform in school. *Publication of the Institute for Family Studies.* Retrieved January 26, 2019, from https://ifstudies.org/blog/the-adoptive-difference-new-evidence-on-how-adopted-children-perform-in-school

Conclusion

What have we learned within the last 30 years about complex childhood trauma, child development mediated by trauma, and Developmental Trauma Disorder (DTD) while working with internationally adopted post-institutionalized children? The outcome of research in the field of international adoption is to attain an adequate understanding of DTD in IAPI children and provide the proper means of scaffolding former institutional residents to be productive, self-sufficient, emotionally stable, and law-abiding members of our society. What are the lessons we have learned so far??

First, merely removing a young child from an environment of neglect and deprivation is not a guarantee of positive outcomes. Repetitive traumatization in human relationships from early childhood mediates the child development by creating distortions and impairments that are difficult, and at times impossible, to remediate. Trauma causes distortions in the important abilities to form social relations, advance cognitively, and behave within socially acceptable norms.

Second, children who were abandoned by their biological parents, spent their earliest months and years in an orphanage, and then adopted by strangers from abroad, tend to develop a certain set of behaviors ("post-orphanage syndrome") that are merely survival skills formed to handle their new environment. These patterns of behavior are often misinterpreted as oppositional defiant behaviors, mood disorders, hyperactivity, or even as autistic spectrum disorder; therefore, the children are mistakenly treated with ineffective behavioral management techniques or medication. Proper understanding of the consequences of a profound complex childhood trauma is required for successful rehabilitation and remediation of international adoptees.

Third, strangely or not, the age of adoption doesn't entirely correlate with the positive results. The damage done prenatal or in the first most formative years of life too often has lifelong consequences. It seemed intuitive to assume that the younger a child is adopted, the better chances there are to remold him or her and remediate the damage done to victims of complex childhood trauma. Alas, the experience failed to confirm this assumption. In the case of irreversible neurological damage, no matter how early the corrective course began, the positive outcome was equally difficult or even impossible to gain. It is true that the younger the child at the time of adoption, the more time may be spent in rehabilitation, sparing more abuse and suffering, but the results may not match the efforts. A lot of statistical data, not merely clinical experience, confirmed that children adopted at as early as several months old may still become deeply troubled youngsters in their teenage years and young adulthood.

Fourth, soon after internationally adopted children from third world countries arrive, they enter the most advanced educational systems in the world. Coping with school issues and competing against middle-class native speakers of English, constitutes still another link in the long chain of traumatization. For the majority of international adoptees adopted at or close to school-age, a regular education program must be replaced by remediation. Before these children join the mainstream classroom, they need to be remediated to be able to take advantage of a regular curriculum.

Fifth, internationally adopted children have experienced the most severe form of neglect, which mediates their development for many years of their post-adoption life. Still, the human mind and body have immense resources and resilience. The effect of social-induced trauma environment is influential but not final: to some extent even organic injury may be fully or partially corrected, depending on the degree of damage and the rehabilitation methods. International adoptees need therapeutic parenting in the family, intensive and focused remediation at school, and highly specialized mental health services, if needed, in the community. IAPI children challenge us to find better treatments for the rehabilitation and remediation and to work on expending the boundaries of restoration for them and other children afflicted by trauma.

* * *

Everything written about international adoption can be roughly defined as inspirational, instructional, or research/clinical. The first category is meant to encourage; it offers a positive message that everything is going to be fine and is, by far, the most satisfying read. The second category is written for the parents and professionals to promote common sense understanding of issues in international adoption and offer an instructional "know-how" to address these issues. The writers are often parents themselves and professionals who have been in the trenches of this field. A physician normally does not deal with healthy people, and adoptive families with no issues will not knock at the door of a psychological office. Therefore, often the authors of the instructional books have skewed and off-centered viewpoints like those of any other "crisis intervention" workers'. The third category of publications are research-based articles, books, or book chapters written by specialists in different disciplines, mostly mental health professionals. Only a few of the researches have personal long-term clinical experience working with international adoptees in the family, hospital, and school context. The instruments they are using are designed and approbated on general population and often rather questionable in relation to such an unusual population as international adoptees. In short, there is not an "ideal" perspective on the controversially understood, emotionally charged, and politically sensitive human endeavor called "international adoption."

To quote the famous movie line, "You can't handle the truth!" However, not only can we handle the truth, but we must. Because a rose-colored view painted by "those in the business" often leads to disasters: mental, emotional, and financial. Because some people should not adopt, and some children are better off not being adopted. Because, contrary to an optimistic stand, in real life, love doesn't conquer all.

After a 30-year involvement, what are my attitude, feelings, and opinion on international adoption? The simple answer is, it depends.

I believe that forming realistic expectations, having as much preparedness as possible, and mobilizing all available resources could give a prospective adoptive parent a chance, not a guarantee, of a successful international adoption. I believe that adoption is not an event, but a process. I consider adoption as a two-way street: like marriage, it takes two to make a family; therefore, characteristics of parents are as important as the attributes of their child. And we have to add what is known as a "social context"—a mixture of culture, language, race, collective expectations, attitudes, and pre-conceptions—to this already complex picture.

I think that if a person enters this incredibly risky speedway in the right vehicle, with a cool, calm, and collected spirit, true knowledge of the "traffic," and a firm resolution to make this journey, then Lady Luck will be kind to this driver.

No one can predict what happens in international adoption tomorrow or 20 years down the road. There are still many thousands of orphans worldwide and many couples, individuals, and families wishing to welcome parentless children from overseas into their homes. Although international adoption has never been a solution for the world's orphan crisis, it is a way out for an individual child, and this chance makes the world better, one person at a time. Our collective knowledge and experience with international adoption is our united/shared treasure that helps us with the process and the end result. International adoption is alive, changing its geography, procedures, demands, and the character of its participants. My sincere hope is that my clinical and research experience reflected in this book will be a fitting contribution to this decent human endeavor.

Appendix 1
Developmental Trauma Disorder Questionnaire for the Parents of Internationally Adopted Post-Institutionalized Children

Please read the statements that follow carefully and specify if, to the best of your knowledge, the child has experienced trauma described as follows:

I. Total abandonment at birth by biological parents

    1. Definitely no

    2. It is not known

    3. It is likely (alleged or suspected, but not documented)

    4. Definitely yes

    Please indicate the age as 0–3, 3–6, 6–9, 9-up?

Comments:

II. Repeated abandonment (frequently left alone for many hours and days) during early childhood

    1. Definitely no

    2. It is not known

    3. It is likely (alleged or suspected, but not documented)

    4. Definitely yes

    Please indicate the age as 0–3, 3–6, 6–9, 9-up?

Comments:

III. Death, severe mental/physical impairment, or prolong unavailability of the principal caregiver due to alcohol or drug abuse

    1. Definitely no

    2. It is not known

    3. It is likely (alleged or suspected, but not documented)

    4. Definitely yes

    Please indicate the age as 0–3, 3–6, 6–9, 9-up?

Comments:

IV. Repeated change/separation from caregivers due to multiple placements

1. Definitely no

2. It is not known

3. It is likely (alleged or suspected, but not documented)

4. Definitely yes

Please indicate the age as 0–3, 3–6, 6–9, 9-up?

Comments:

V. Failed adoption or foster care (disruption) in the native country or in the US

1. Definitely no

2. It is not known

3. It is likely (alleged or suspected, but not documented)

4. Definitely yes

Please indicate the age as 0–3, 3–6, 6–9, 9-up?

Comments:

VI. Extreme physical discomfort: hunger, cold, heat, dehydration, etc.

1. Definitely no

2. It is not known

3. It is likely (alleged or suspected, but not documented)

4. Definitely yes

Please indicate the age as 0–3, 3–6, 6–9, 9-up?

Comments:

VII. Extreme neglect of the child's basic physical and emotional needs, if reported or documented

1. Definitely no

2. It is not known

3. It is likely (alleged or suspected, but not documented)

4. Definitely yes

Please indicate the age as 0–3, 3–6, 6–9, 9-up?

Comments:

VIII. Physical abuse: beating, torturing, etc., by caregivers

1. Definitely no

2. It is not known

3. It is likely (alleged or suspected, but not documented)

4. Definitely yes

Please indicate the age as 0–3, 3–6, 6–9, 9-up?

Comments:

IX. Witnessing violence, physical assault, murder, beating, drinking, and/or sexual orgies

1. Definitely no

2. It is not known

3. It is likely (alleged or suspected, but not documented)

4. Definitely yes

Please indicate the age as 0–3, 3–6, 6–9, 9-up?

Comments:

X. Chronic illness, physical impairment, injury, or dysmorphic features (e.g., cleft palate)

1. Definitely no

2. It is not known

3. It is likely (alleged or suspected, but not documented)

4. Definitely yes

Please indicate the age as 0–3, 3–6, 6–9, 9-up?

Comments:

XI. Placement in an institution (orphanage or hospital) and transferred between institutions

1. Definitely no

2. It is not known

3. It is likely (alleged or suspected, but not documented)

4. Definitely yes

Please indicate the age as 0–3, 3–6, 6–9, 9-up?

Comments:

XII. All kinds of abuse by peers (from bulling to rape) in the orphanage

1. Definitely no

2. It is not known

3. It is likely (alleged or suspected, but not documented)

4. Definitely yes

Please indicate the age as 0–3, 3–6, 6–9, 9-up?

Comments:

XIII. Adoption to foreign country: sudden loss of language, racial identity, and cultural and physical environment

1. Definitely no

2. It is not known

3. It is likely (alleged or suspected, but not documented)

4. Definitely yes

Please indicate the age as 0–3, 3–6, 6–9, 9-up?

Comments:

XIV. Adjustment to new social, cultural, and physical environment: family life, new ethnic or racial community

1. Definitely no

2. It is not known

3. It is likely (alleged or suspected, but not documented)

4. Definitely yes

Could you indicate the age as 0–3, 3–6, 6–9, 9-up?

Comments:

XV. Negative experiences at school in the new country

1. Definitely no

2. It is not known

3. It is likely (alleged or suspected, but not documented)

4. Definitely yes

Please indicate the age as 0–3, 3–6, 6–9, 9-up?

Comments:

XVI. Traumatic experiences within the adoptive family: death, severe illness, life-threatening accidents (e.g., fire, car crash), divorce, home violence, community carnage, frequent change of place of residents, etc.

    1. Definitely no   3. It is likely (alleged or suspected, but not documented)

    2. It is not known   4. Definitely yes

                           Please indicate the age as 0–3, 3–6, 6–9, 9-up?

Comments:

XVII. Traumatic experiences related to race, ethnic belonging, or national identity of the adopted child in relation to his or her adoptive family and community.

    1. Definitely no   3. It is likely (alleged or suspected, but not documented)

    2. It is not known   4. Definitely yes

                           Please indicate the age as 0–3, 3–6, 6–9, 9-up?

Comments:

XVIII. Other traumatic events. Please specify:

Appendix 2

Sample of Referral Questions and Psychological Tools Used in Bilingual Screening of Newly Arrived Internationally Adopted Post-Institutionalized Children

This psychoeducational screening and related consultation were requested by Dr. H., superintendent for L. Central School District, at the request of Mr. and Mrs. F. for their son Dmitry, a 7-year-and-5-month-old boy who was adopted from a Russian orphanage and brought to the USA three weeks prior to this assessment. The referral parties are interested in knowing the following:

- Dmitry's current developmental status in terms of his cognitive, language, and social skills/adaptive behavior.
- Whether Dmitry has specific educational handicapping conditions that may prevent him from acquiring academic skills at an age-appropriate level due to has diagnosis of a genetic-based disorder (albinism).
- Dmitry's academic readiness for a mainstream US school curriculum.
- Whether Dmitry needs academic remediation that goes beyond the range of expected problems related to this international adoption (e.g., second-language acquisition and social adjustment). If so, in which academic subjects?
- The most appropriate educational setting for Dmitry now (spring/ summer of 2017) and in the fall of 2017. The most appropriate educational classification, academic placement, level of instruction, supportive services, classroom accommodations, and test modifications if Dmitry needs a modified learning environment.

In order to answer the above presented referral questions, the following set of tests and clinical procedures were used:

- Review of the original adoption-related legal and medical documentation.
- Intake conference with adoptive parents using the **Developmental Trauma Disorder Scale.**
- Clinical observations of the child's behavior and social interactions during testing using **Quick Neurological Screening Test—3R**

(a screening tool for "soft" neurological signs in observable behavior) and **NEPSY-II** Guidelines and Behavior Observations Tables.

- **Universal Nonverbal Intelligence Test-2 (UNIT-2)**—a standardized test to determine intellectual potential without direct language involvement.
- **Woodcock-Johnson Psychoeducational Battery, IV, Tests of Cognitive Abilities**—selected *nonverbal* tests.
- **The Bender Visual-Motor Gestalt Test**, second edition, and samples of handwriting and drawings.
- **NEPSY-II** (developmental neuropsychological assessment)—selected tests for grapho-motor proficiency.
- **Bilingual Verbal Ability Tests** (Russian form)—standardized tests of cognitive/academic language in Russian.
- The Luria Language Processing Test (LLPT, 1996 revision, in the Russian language)—a non-standardized test for evaluating communicative fluency/pragmatics and reasoning/comprehension in the Russian language.
- **Woodcock-Johnson III, Tests of Achievement**—math tests only, translated into Russian.
- An estimation of academic skills according to the Russian Federation official curriculum for the first through fourth grades (Olma Press instructional material—Moscow, 2010) in reading, writing, and general fund of information.

A Statement About the Language of Assessment and the Use of Standardized Tests

This is the first formal developmental, psychological, and educational evaluation given to Dmitry in the US. The evaluation was performed by a licensed psychologist with native fluency and proper certification for assessments in the Russian language, with specialization in the field of international adoption and extensive experience evaluating children adopted from the countries of Eastern Europe[1].

The language of the assessment is a rather unique and a critically important factor in the evaluation of internationally adopted children. (For more discussion, please see B. Gindis (2009), Neuropsychological Assessment of Internationally Adopted Children: What to Expect? *The Family Focus* (FRUA, Washington, DC) vol. XV, no. 1, pp. 4–8[2]) At the time of this assessment, Dmitry's dominant mode of communication and literacy was Russian. All verbal tests were administered in Russian and all testing instructions were given in Russian. Still other psychological tests and clinical procedures were administered through nonverbal means, requiring no verbal input or output. All standardized tests and behavior rating scales were administered according to their specific manuals. However, these tests and behavior scales are standardized instruments with limited validity for this foreign-born child with an atypical cultural background. Thus, according to *the Standards for Educational and Psychological Testing* , developed jointly by the American Psychological Association the American Educational Research Association, and the National Council on Measurement in Education[3], a strictly normative interpretation of the test scores or behavior ratings was not possible due to deviations from standard procedures to accommodate bilingual issues. Therefore, all quantitative test results in this report should be considered an approximated estimation of Dmitry's current psychological and educational functioning rather than a measurement; these numerical data are offered as a baseline for comparison for future assessments, and performance on all standardized tests should be interpreted as "no less than."

Notes

1. see www.bgcenter.com
2. www.bgcenter.com/BGPublications/NeuropsychologicalAssessment.htm
3. www.apa.org/science/standards.html

Appendix 3

Sample of Referral Questions and Psychoeducational Tests/Clinical Procedures Used for a Comprehensive Combined Neuropsychological, Developmental, and Educational Assessment of Internationally Adopted Post-Institutionalized Children

This evaluation was requested by Mr. and Mrs. C. for their 9-year-old son Theodor, adopted from a Poland orphanage four years ago. The following questions were formulated and/or approved by the referring party:

- What is Theodor's current developmental status in terms of his cognitive, language, and social/emotional functioning?
- What are Theodor's academic strengths and weaknesses in the age-appropriate grade curriculum, and what is the baseline to compare his academic progress over the next 12–18 months?
- Does Theodor have a sufficient cognitive/academic language base for mastering the curriculum at age- and grade-appropriate levels? What is his level of communicative fluency and pragmatics?
- What is the nature of Theodor's behavioral/emotional problems? Does Theodor have organic-based impairments, developmental delays, or psychological disorders underlying his current behavioral and emotional issues at home and in school? In this context, what are his differential diagnoses in the social/emotional domain?
- What is the nature of Theodor's educational needs? Specifically, does he have any educationally handicapping conditions that may prevent him from acquiring literacy skills at an age-appropriate level?
- To what extent does Theodor's developmental history contribute to his current adaptive functioning, and how can this factor be addressed therapeutically?
- How can Theodor's learning and social issues be effectively addressed in school and in the family in a way that will positively impact his learning and emotional well-being? What remedial educational methodologies and therapeutic behavioral interventions are needed to address Theodor's current academic and behavioral/emotional needs? If Theodor needs a modified learning environment, what would be the most appropriate educational setting, level of instruction, supportive services, classroom accommodations, and test modifications for him?

In order to respond to the above presented referral questions, the following set of tests and clinical procedures were used in this assessment (standardized tests and behavior scales are presented in **bold**).

Domain: Developmental History

- Review of the adoption-related medical and legal documentation
- Review of school documentation, including the most current IEP
- An initial interview with the parents using the NEPSY-II Child Developmental History and the **Developmental Trauma Disorder Scale**

Domain: Adaptive Behavior/Skills and Social/Emotional Functioning

Clinical observations of behavior and social interaction during testing using **NEPSY-II Guidelines and Behavior Observations Tables and Quick Neurological Screening Test-3, Revised**—a screening test for "soft" neurological signs in observable behavior.

Interview the parents and school personnel using the following:

- **Devereux Behavior Rating Scale,** Parent and Teacher Forms (psychopathology of behavior)
- **Adaptive Behavior Assessment System 3, Parent Form** (general adaptive behavior)
- DSM-5 Generic Checklist of Child Depression Disorder Symptoms
- **DSM-5-based ADHD Symptoms Checklist, Parent and Teacher Form**
- **Social Responsiveness Scale, 2nd Edition** (Parent and Teacher Forms)—a standardized measure of reciprocity in social behavior
- Sensory Integration Disorder Survey for Parents
- **Disturbance of Attachment Clinical Interview (ages 5 to 12 version)**

Clinical interviews with Theodor using the following:

- Projective Questionnaire and Incomplete Sentences Blank
- **Revised Children's Manifest Anxiety Scale, 2nd Edition**—self-report of anxiety symptoms
- **Affect Recognition and Theory of Mind subtests from NEPSY-II**
- **Emotional acuity test from the NECOG battery**

Domain: General Intellectual Functioning and Specific Cognitive Processes/Skills

- **Woodcock-Johnson Psychoeducational Battery IV, Tests of Cognitive Abilities (WJ-IV-C)**—a standardized test of general cognitive abilities and processes

- NEPSY-II (developmental neuropsychological assessment)—selected tests for specific psychological functions
- Wechsler Intelligence Scale for Children, 5th Edition (WISC-5)—a standardized test of general cognitive abilities and processes
- Neurocognitive Assessment Battery—SNS Vital Signs—a computerized measure of complex attention, processing speed, response inhibition, and executive functioning.
- Behavior Rating Inventory for Executive Function (BRIEF)—a measure of self-regulation and goal-directed behavior.

Domain: Language—Cognitive/Academic and Social Aspects

- Woodcock-Johnson IV, Tests of Oral Language—a measure of cognitive/academic language
- NEPSY-II (developmental neuropsychological assessment)—selected tests on language comprehension and oro-motor proficiency
- Social Language Development Test—a standardized measure of pragmatics and social language skills

Domain: Academic Knowledge and Skills

- Woodcock-Johnson IV, Tests of Achievement—subtests relevant to the instructional curriculum for the appropriate age and grade

Domain: Alcohol-Related Neurodevelopmental Disorder (ARND) Diagnostic Procedure

4-Digit Diagnostic Guide for Fetal Alcohol Spectrum Disorders, 3rd Edition (FASD Diagnostic and Prevention Network, Seattle WA, 2004), including computer-based facial features analysis as a clinical procedure for the differential diagnosis procedure of ARND

Index

Note: Page numbers in bold indicate a table on the corresponding page.

For Product Safety Concerns and Information please contact our
EU representative GPSR@taylorandfrancis.com Taylor & Francis
Verlag GmbH, Kaufingerstraße 24, 80331 München, Germany